Busting Your Butt and Gut

MINIMIZING YOUR MAXIMUM AREAS

Marty Tuley

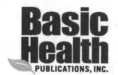

Basic Health
PUBLICATIONS, INC.

The information contained in this book is based upon the research and personal and professional experiences of the author. It is not intended as a substitute for consulting with your physician or other healthcare provider. Any attempt to diagnose and treat an illness should be done under the direction of a healthcare professional.

The publisher does not advocate the use of any particular healthcare protocol but believes the information in this book should be available to the public. The publisher and author are not responsible for any adverse effects or consequences resulting from the use of the suggestions, preparations, or procedures discussed in this book. Should the reader have any questions concerning the appropriateness of any procedures or preparation mentioned, the author and the publisher strongly suggest consulting a professional healthcare advisor.

Basic Health Publications, Inc.
28812 Top of the World Drive
Laguna Beach, CA 92651
949-715-7327 · www.basichealthpub.com

Library of Congress Cataloging-in-Publication Data

Tuley, Marty.
    Busting your butt and gut : minimizing your maximum areas / Marty Tuley.
        p. cm.
    Includes index.
    ISBN 978-1-59120-208-0
  1. Physical fitness. 2. Buttocks. 3. Abdomen. 4. Reducing exercises. I. Title.

    RA781.T838   2008
    613.7'1—dc22

                                                            2008016045

Illustrations on pages 8 and 9 from LifeART/MediClip, copyright © 2008 Wolters Kluwer Health, Inc.—Lippincott Williams & Wilkins. All rights reserved.

Editor: John Anderson
Typesetting/Graphic Design: Gary A. Rosenberg & Terry Wiscovitch
Cover Designer: Mike Stromberg

Printed in the United States of America

10   9   8   7   6   5   4   3   2   1

Praise for Marty Tuley's

Get Off Your Ass!

A book I can recommend without hesitation,
with "both of my thumbs" up!

—WILLIAM LLEWELLYN, OWNER OF MOLECULAR NUTRITION

Tactlessness aside, it's hard to argue with his logic or
the advice [Tuley] offers throughout the book.

—JOHN HANC, *NEW YORK NEWSDAY*

Get Off Your Ass hits you right between the eyes
with a dose of reality . . . and that's much needed in
American society where fraud and deception dominate
the most noble of industries . . . the fitness industry.
Marty speaks to the reader as if he is right there
in the reader's corner, acting as a coach, a trainer,
and an educator. No doubt this book will change lives.

—PHIL KAPLAN, *MIND & MUSCLE FITNESS HOUR RADIO SHOW*

Marty doesn't beat around the bush and he is the
only guy that can tell me to "Get off *my* ass,"
whose ass I won't kick.

—LANA, OWNER OF LANA'S EGG WHITES

Get Off Your Ass!

Marty Tuley is the best kind of iconoclast: He knows
the conventional as well as the unconventional,
and boils it down to the simplest admonition:
"Dude, get it in gear!" He combines logic and passion
in equal doses, and that's an unbeatable combination.

—LOU SCHULER, AUTHOR OF *THE BOOK OF MUSCLE*
AND *THE TESTOSTERONE ADVANTAGE PLAN*

Marty Tuley . . . on one hand . . . a gritty, over the top,
in your face, tell it like it is muscle head akin to a drill sergeant.
On the other . . . a witty, charming, handsome, sincere young
man with a *compelling message,* who truly enjoys nothing
more than being the *catalyst* that changes lives.

—TAMMY PETERSEN, AMERICAN ACADEMY OF HEALTH AND FITNESS

CONTENTS

ACKNOWLEDGMENTS

Thanks to my son, Ryeki, born July 25, 2005. I had no idea.

Thanks, Lovena, for your support, your character, your friendship, and your love.

Thanks, Mom. You're the pillar of the family.

Thanks, little sister. You've always been there.

Thanks, Dimitri. You're continually showing me what love and family really are.

Thanks, Belchers. The best people I've ever known.

Thanks, Uncle Jim. I consider your teachings often.

Thanks, Neesha. I'm grateful you touched my life.

Thanks, Blitz. You're *still* reminding me daily that life is simple and simple is all that matters.

Thanks, Hauck Brothers. Two pioneering spirits who left Holland in 1749, threw caution to the wind, and decided that without risk there can be no reward. I hope at least a drop of their blood courses through my veins.

FOREWORD

If you've decided to read this book, you're undoubtedly searching for a way to slim down and shape up two specific areas of your anatomy. You won't be disappointed, but you might be surprised. By following the incredible program in *Busting Your Butt and Gut,* you'll get results that you've only dreamed about in the past. You'll also get something far better than a dramatic change in your physique: as you reshape your body, you'll be reshaping your attitude, your health, and your life.

This book, like Marty Tuley's fitness philosophy, is guided by three key principles. The first is information: you need to know exactly what to do—and exactly how to do it—in order to achieve the desired results. When it comes to shaping and strengthening your glutes and abs, what are the best exercises, and how are they performed? The information is all here. What you hold in your hand is a roadmap to success. If you follow the directions, you'll arrive at the desired destination. It's that simple.

The second key principle is integrity: Marty is a breath of fresh air—a fitness expert who can always be counted on to tell it like it is, no holds barred. He's not afraid to confront the truth, no matter how unwelcome or uncomfortable it may be. If you're looking for someone who will encourage you to accept mediocrity, or allow you to settle for good excuses instead of your best effort, keep looking. If, on the other hand, you're in search of a coach and a mentor who will challenge you to develop the dedication, discipline, and consistency that you must have to succeed, Marty's your man.

The third principle upon which *Busting Your Butt and Gut* is based is inspiration: it's what we're all searching for, and yet we rarely find it. Even the best and most accurate information won't help you if you aren't inspired to take action. Marty is one of the most motivated—and motivating—individuals I know. Why? He's not only living what he's teaching, he's loving it. He also wants you to live it and love it. It's impossible to read this book without thinking, "Yes, I can do this. I can succeed!"

If you follow the program, you will succeed. It's straightforward and simple. But don't confuse "simple" with "easy." The program is simple in that it isn't difficult to understand or to implement, and it requires no special facilities or equipment. No gym membership? No problem. You don't need high-tech weight machines, cardio equipment, or even an exercise ball to complete the program. As Marty says, all you need is a pulse and an attitude. That attitude will come in handy when you accept the fact that the *Busting Your Butt and Gut* program isn't easy or effortless. You will work and you will sweat—that's how you'll know you're accomplishing your goals. On the journey to success, there are no shortcuts.

The good news is that by following Marty's program, the journey to success can be broken down into small, manageable steps. Twenty minutes a day, six days a week. The exercises are designed to give you the maximum return on every single minute of your workout, so that in terms of time and effort, you get the biggest bang for your buck.

Every minute you invest in the program is an investment in yourself—in your self-confidence, your appearance, your health, and even your life. Marty Tuley is an expert you can trust. *Busting Your Butt and Gut* is a program you can believe in. Now, all you have to do is trust and believe in yourself.

—Rallie McAllister, M.D., MPH, MSEH

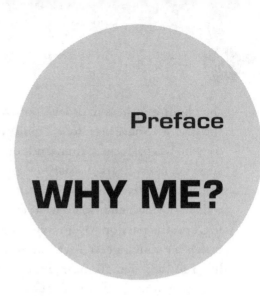

Preface

WHY ME?

*"Believe one who has proved it.
Believe an expert."*

—VIRGIL (70 B.C. TO 19 B.C.)

I AM OFTEN ASKED, "Were *you* ever fat?" The answer is "no." I have never been obese or "battled the bulge," at least not in the way most people associate the weight loss wars. Instead, I started pumping iron at the tender age of fourteen and have never stopped. I have been happily and monogamously married to exercise for twenty-five years! How about that for dedication? Does that *disqualify* me as a fitness or weight loss expert? Does that make it impossible for me to understand the issues faced by those who are battling obesity? Am I disqualified simply because I lack their real life experience of being fat and out of shape?

People have asked me, "How can you know the emotions associated with the momentous task of changing ones health and fitness and establishing new habits?" True, I've never battled such demons, but from an early age, I established fitness as a habit. I based my success on establishing habit, *not* physically measurable goals. That's a key point, because every model I am aware of starts with the premise of setting up the goal of some form of physical, measurable change. And those models have been and are continuing to fail *miserably*!

It is unrealistic to believe that an individual must suffer or experience the plight of others in order to provide help. Are the good lawyers only the ones who have been found guilty of a felony? Would you prefer a doctor who has performed thousands of open-heart surgeries or one that has suffered from heart disease? Does your dentist have crooked, yellow teeth? I have never been fat, but *that* is what qualifies me! I've done it—I've walked the path and I *know* what it takes. I have the experience, the training, and the passion to show you the journey. I've never been fat, which makes me your biggest asset. You're about to embark on the fight of your life. Your opponent is mean, nasty, and tough. In this fight, you're going to take a punch or two, but you've got an experienced cornerman to help you.

Chapter 1

CHANGE YOUR LIFE!

"The person who makes a success of living is one who sees his goal steadily and aims for it unswervingly. That is dedication."

—CECIL B. DeMILLE (1881–1959)

Your Armor, Your Shield, and Your Sword

WHEN I AM ASKED TO DESCRIBE the most important keys to the lifestyle of health and fitness, I respond without hesitation that they are dedication, discipline and consistency. Forget everything you think you know about fitness. The "secret" lies in the understanding and application of those three words.

Surprised? The secrets to success are not about your total daily calories or how many times you're exercising per week. It's not about what gym you belong to or what program you're currently following. It's not about your age, your gender, or how busy your day is. It's about a mind-set. It's about change, about getting off your ass and feeling good about it. It's about putting your head down and forging ahead through the storm of life with your bow breaking the waves and your sails corralling the wind. It's about not taking the easy road—the road most traveled. Don't go there because it's a highway backed up and overcrowded with people lost with the map right in their hands. I am not talking about exercise at this point. If you want to accomplish *anything* worthwhile, you'd better get to know the words *dedication, discipline,* and *consistency.*

Discipline is your armor. Dave Draper, author of *Brother Iron, Sister Steel*, says this of discipline, "I go nowhere good without it." Many treat and see discipline as a burden or something to shy away from. Don't confuse discipline with obsession: discipline enriches your life, while obsession devours it. Do not fear discipline. Wear it as a knight wears his armor—it is your first line of defense.

Dedication is your shield, an extension of your armor of discipline. If you're dedicated to something, and people use the word to describe your action, then you're running at a whole different level. And *dedicated* is not a word people throw around easily. If you've been described as "dedicated," then you're probably half a step off your ass already. .

Consistency is your sword. Drop it and the battle is lost. Discipline and dedication are your defense, but consistency is your offense. A sword is heavy: the weight makes it difficult and demanding to wield, but wield it you must. Keep consistency tightly in your hands.

Forget about asking what the world can offer—start taking what you deserve! Remember, you are not a fanatic if you've decided that exercise and eating right are going to be a part of your life. You are not selfish or self-centered for realizing that care of yourself is the first step to taking care of others. You are not egocentric if hitting the gym is part of your daily ritual. I am not asking you to become obsessive, self-centered, or one-dimensional. Caring about how you look and feel is not fanatical, but it does take dedication, discipline, and consistency. Three better allies you'll not find.

"You may be disappointed if you fail,
but you are doomed if you don't try."
—BEVERLY SILLS (B. 1929)

You Will Fail!

You will fail. How about that? Yes, that's right, I said "fail." It's unavoidable, so don't get discouraged. I am not saying don't try—I'm saying never *quit*! People fail every day. We are not perfect and nobody does everything "out of the gate" without trips or stumbles. We fall and we fall a lot. We also fail a lot, but how many of us dust off our knees, get back up, and push our way right back to the front lines? Not many and not enough. Like a boxer, you've got to learn to take a punch.

Failure is part of life. More often than not, we must fail in order to learn, and they're often hard lessons to learn indeed. Failure hurts: it leaves scars, both visible and invisible. And often the scars from failure never heal, but instead linger throughout our lifetime as open sores or infected wounds, causing pain way beyond their first infliction. The wounds never heal because they are never treated. These battle wounds are like an unfinished painting, a masterpiece that is started but never completed.

Finish your masterpiece. Dust off you knees, get your paintbrushes back out, and storm the front lines. Realize you are going to fail, but resolve to yourself to *never* quit. Individuals fail every day, but they continuing waging the war, never quitting. That's the silver lining in the reality of failure. Amassing scars but no sores, no open wounds, no untreated injuries—just reminders of hard times, hard battles, and hard decisions. What is the hardest decision and choice of all? Deciding that failing is an unavoidable outcome of trying but then choosing to *never* quit!

> *"I have often wished I had time to cultivate modesty . . .*
> *But I am too busy thinking about myself."*
> —EDITH SITWELL (1887–1964)

"You Can't Polish a Turd"

Individuals—teachers, neighbors, a co-worker, counselor, a boyhood friend, or a cousin—touch us and influence us in various ways throughout our lives. Some affect us only briefly, while others, like family members, may provide insight and guidance for much our lives. For me, such an individual is my Uncle Jim. From an early age, I found Uncle Jim to be an individual for whom I had deep respect. He is kind, fair, and driven, and I listen with ears wide open whenever he speaks. Uncle Jim has provided me with many simple, precise, and thoughtful bits of wisdom. His advice is easy to remember, difficult to apply, and even harder to adhere to.

I've heard the saying "You can't polish a turd" from others, but it's a phrase I associate with my Uncle Jim and him alone. Besides, words are just words unless their source also happens to be representative of a character we can admire, unless those who utter them also practice what they preach. My Uncle Jim is such a man, a natural-born philosopher.

Fitness is like philosophy—we understand it and recognize it, but we struggle with the implementation. We know how we *should* be, but seemingly lack the resolution to achieve it. This is where my Uncle Jim's words of wisdom come to mind. "Quick fixes" are feeble tries at self-change that buff our outside but leave our character open and unchanged. Quick fixes are turd polishers.

Quit polishing the turd! It's like you're waxing the car, worrying about the paint job, and all the while it's sitting on blocks with a blown engine. Quit buying fancy curtains to hang on your run-down house. Harsh? Maybe, but you and I both know it is true. We live in the age of instant *anything*! Twenty-four hours a day, seven days a week, what do you want? It's there, available, at our fingertips. If you've got the money, it's yours. Sound familiar? We're all susceptible to the fortunes (and misfortunes) of the economic juggernaut America has become, but we can no longer use ignorance as an excuse.

Our hard work and drive as a culture have made goods accessible and cheap, but in some respects our economic fortune has cost us patience, pride, and self-respect. Many have chosen liposuction over self-control, stomach staples in place of restraint, and "nips and tucks" in place of a fitness routine. We walk paths and make choices that place our lives in danger, ironically gambling with our health in order to look . . . healthy. It's a dangerous paradox to be sure, all done in a vain attempt to "polish our turds."

Let's be clear, the Butt & Gut Program is *not* an "end all and be all" program, but it's also not a turd polisher. It is one step of many that you will take over the course of your life to preserve, improve, or even repair your health and fitness. There are no single programs or specific diets that you can undertake and uphold your entire life. They just don't exist. Instead, I hope that the Butt & Gut Program teaches you the *real* secret—eat a consistent, balanced diet, exercise regularly, and quit polishing your turd!

> *"A sound mind in a sound body is a short but full
> description of a happy state in this world."*
> —JOHN LOCKE (1632–1704)

Anatomy—The Basics

Before we get to the Butt & Gut Program, I want to give you some foundational insights into anatomy and physiology. I wrote *Busting Your Butt and Gut* with two areas of the body as my leading consideration. For most people, excess weight collects on your derriere and in your midsection. There are exceptions, of course, but at least initially most of the weight gain that we don't want piles up on the butt and gut.

However, I am not going to bore you with too much of the technical physiology of your butt and gut. It's just not that important that you know where a particular muscle originates or where its point of insertion is located. Neither is it important that you have an understanding of fast-twitch muscles fibers and slow-twitch muscle fibers or their roles. Many experts, trainers, and authors overemphasize this topic, placing *way* too much importance on the average person's need to understand muscle physiology. More often than not, this attempt at education (it's really just book "filler") results in confused and overwhelmed students. You're interested in changing your health and fitness, not in earning a degree in kinesiology or physiology. This section provides you with the basic physiology of the areas that this book discusses, your butt and gut.

"There's no easy way out. If there were, I would have bought it.
And believe me, it would be one of my favorite things!"
—OPRAH WINFREY (B. 1954)

She's Got the Booty, He's Got the Belly

There are several differences between the genders. In fact, sometimes it's difficult to even see any likenesses between men and women. One notable difference to add to the list is how men and women spread their excess weight. It shouldn't come as a surprise that men and women carry extra, unwanted pounds in different areas of the body. Just look around. Men develop a "beer belly" and women tend to develop "saddlebags."

Why do men and women carry their respective excesses in this way? I am not sure anyone knows and, maybe more importantly, I am not sure it matters. But it appears that nature, evolution, God, or whatever other power has designed us in this manner. However, the geography of our fat storage isn't that important. It's the means and mechanism of fat's exodus from our physiques that should most concern us. In other words, men and women carry fat differently, but we gain it and lose it in much the same manner.

A muscle cell needs roughly thirty-eight calories a day to preserve its existence in your body. Why is that significant? Because a fat cell only needs a whopping two calories! What that means is that a fat cell is much, much easier for your body to keep and add. This is why it's rather easy to get fat and typically hard as hell to get back in shape. This is also why when you "crash" diet by substantially reducing your total calories, you may get lighter but also possibly *fatter*. Your weight decreases, but your ratio of fat-to-muscle goes up. Your body may actually discard the high-energy-consuming muscle cells in favor of safeguarding your fat. Eventually, this leads to the dreaded "yo-yo" weight-loss and weight-gain saga. Been there?

Crash diets force your body to choose between a muscle cell, which wants thirty-eight calories, and a fat cell, which needs only two calories. Your body's choice to retain the fat cells is simple economics. Fat cells need less. And since you're eating less (i.e., fewer overall calories) while on your diet, jettisoning the muscle cells seems logical.

This is also why some resistance training is essential, because it forces your body to recognize a need for muscle. Crash dieting without exercise is fitness suicide. You're a ticking time bomb if you're not exercising while you're trying to lose weight. Not exercising slows your metabolism, creating an effective fat-storage machine. This sets you up for a round-trip ticket to your former weight and almost guarantees that when you return, you'll have new uninvited guests in the form of a larger booty, a larger belly, or both.

You can lose weight—anybody can. The question is can you do it in a way that won't have you right back at the same bus station with a few more bags? The answer is yes, but it comes with understanding how and why. You have to understand the roles that fat and muscle play in your body, the dance they perform and the importance of the music you select. In other words, learn to make your body work for you, not against you.

Nothing is more important than resistance training for both successful weight loss and for keeping the weight off. Do not place calorie cutting or excessive cardiovascular training first in order of importance for weight loss. You may shrink your belly or booty quicker, but it will be short-lived and the quickly savored success will leave as hurriedly as it arrived. Let's lose your booty and your belly, but let's do it the first time. And let's do it *one* time.

> *"Human beings, by changing the inner attitudes of their minds, can change the outer aspects of their lives."*
> —WILLIAM JAMES (1842–1910)

Scientifically Speaking

The glutes are a large muscle area. We often refer to this area as the butt, booty, the rear, derriere, backside, your moneymaker (personal favorite), your junk in the trunk, and a thousand other slang terms. Your abdominals—also a large muscle area—come with a lot fewer colorful, descriptive adjectives. It may have become somewhat trendy to have a fat ass in our society, but a big belly hasn't received the same amount of praise. However, Hollywood is full of surprises and it may be only a matter of time before it somehow turns an excessive belly into something sexy. Meanwhile, let's understand the basic mechanics of these two areas of muscle.

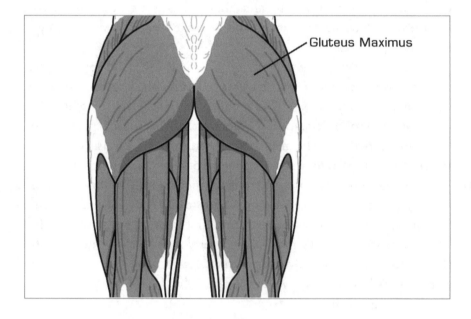

Gluteus Maximus

The glutes are a large, powerful muscle grouping that has been relegated to the role (for most of us) of a seat cushion. (If you could get your ass in shape by sitting on it, most of us would have buns to brag about.) When we discuss the glutes, we're talking about three muscles. The gluteus maximus originates along the pelvic bone crests and attaches to the rear of the femur, which is the large, upper leg bone. The primary role of the gluteus maximus is to move your thigh to the rear, a movement or motion you can do in various ways. Lying beneath the gluteus maximus are the gluteus medius and gluteus minimus. These two muscles also originate from the pelvis, but attach to the side of the femur. Their primary role is to move your leg outward, away from the body.

The abdominals are a grouping of several muscles: the rectus abdominus, transverse abdominus, and the external and internal obliques. The muscles that comprise the abdominals sit on the front and sides of the lower half of the torso. They originate along the rib cage and attach along the pelvis. Together, these muscles perform various roles by bringing the rib cage closer to the pelvis, stabilizing your guts, and rotating your torso.

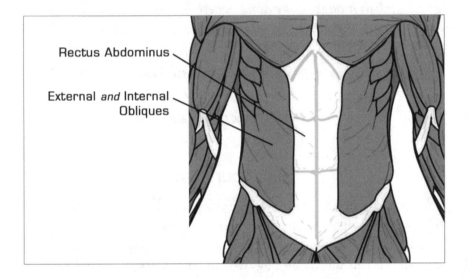

It's important to have a basic understanding of both the location and role of these muscles, because it lays the groundwork for improving your "mind-muscle connection," the link between what your brain says to do and how your muscles first interpret, then respond, to the directions received. Understanding where these muscles are situated and how they function actually improves this process. Exercise itself also strengthens this link: as you exercise, it becomes stronger and more effective, actually increasing the value of your time spent exercising. It's a form of visualization.

Building the mind-muscle connection takes time and patience—it's the nature of the beast—but this is all about baby steps, my friend. Step one: have a *basic* understanding of your anatomy. Step two: begin an exercise program. Together, this becomes the foundation for your success at both starting and maintaining a health and fitness lifestyle. You might gain more attention by sprinting out of the gate, but more often than not you'll also "crash and burn" by doing so. The tortoise wins this race every time.

> *"Perhaps the most valuable result of all education*
> *is the ability to make yourself do the thing you have to do,*
> *when it ought to be done, whether you like it or not;*
> *it is the first lesson that ought to be learned;*
> *and however early a man's training begins,*
> *it is probably the last lesson that*
> *he learns thoroughly."*
>
> —THOMAS H. HUXLEY (1825–1895)

Find Your Path

I realize the daunting nature of improving your health and fitness and I fully recognize the difficulty many of you may have in taking the first precarious steps. Changing your physical self is a daunting proposition indeed. It is this understanding that first motivated me to write *Get Off Your Ass!* and now *Busting Your Butt and Gut.* I want to show everyone how to walk "the path," how to stay on the path, and how to develop an appreciation for the journey. I *know* how much richer your lives will be once you improve your health and fitness.

Don't blame yourself or anyone else for your current physical condition. The simple fact is *this* is where you are. The past is just that—the past. So, leave it there. Let's focus instead on where we're going. I'm reminded of an old saying, "It's not that you spilled the milk. It's how you cleaned it up that matters." The clean-up starts with you, and it starts with a mind-set. You don't have to always be positive. Bad days happen: we have days that we don't feel good, days that we feel depressed, and lazy days when we want to quit and return to our old ways and habits.

But not today, not anymore—from here forward, you will bulldoze your way through. You have it within in you, and you always have had it. In fact, you have it in as great a quantity and quality as the next person, even if you've relegated it to a shoe box in the closet recently. We'll get those old shoes out and wear them out! Break your shoes in. You're just the person for the job.

This is just a step. There are many, *many* more steps to take, so don't kid yourself. Getting and staying in shape is neither quick nor easy, but therein lies the value. We often look for the carrot, and dismiss the value of the gardening and care that went into growing it. Trust me, you'll quickly forget about the carrot, but the work—the hoeing, weeding, tend-

I have written and designed the program in *Busting Your Butt and Gut* for "able-bodied" adults between the ages of 18 and 65—individuals primarily suffering from varying levels of obesity and are simply "out-of-shape" from lack of exercise and overindulgence of food. However, anyone, regardless of their age or perceived state of health, should consult their physician prior to starting regular exercise.

ing, watering, and *the sweat*—will stay with you forever. You'll remember the sacrifice long after you've forgotten what you thought was the reward. Your dedication, your discipline, and your consistency all contribute, create, and foster a little habit, the habit of regular exercise.

Do not take the search for physical fitness lightly. It is a difficult journey, but nonetheless a journey you must undertake. Many take quicker, easier, more dangerous routes. The demand for liposuction and gastric bypass surgery continues to rise. To many people, these medical techniques seem a simple and quick solution to their physical woes. However, these individuals are making the wrong decisions, for mistaken reasons, and suffering for their choice. Modern science is full of miracles—drugs and surgeries for all that ail us—but for all the scientific advances, we forget basic bedrock principles that forge our character and fill our soul. Like a child who's given everything, weight loss surgeries stroke our egos but cannibalize our heart.

There's another way, a course for you to unfold your sails, a journey ripe with failure to be sure, but *long* in reward. It is the path to pride, self-respect, and confidence. It's not hidden; in fact, it's right below your feet. You have unknowingly stepped on it for years, but you have never walked it. It's time to stroll a different path, make a different choice. Here's to you and your first step. Change your life!

Chapter 2

THE IMPORTANCE OF GOOD NUTRITION

"Character is like a tree and reputation like its shadow.
The shadow is what we think of it;
the tree is the real thing."

—ABRAHAM LINCOLN (1809–1865)

BEFORE GETTING TO THE EXERCISE portion of the Butt & Gut Program, it's important to establish a pattern of healthier eating habits. After all, your excess butt and gut didn't just appear out of the blue. In conjunction with your new dedication to exercise, make a commitment to eating foods that are nutritious and will also help you slim down.

What we eat is big news these days. The nation's obesity epidemic has thrust our eating behaviors into the national media. We've made our waistlines front page material, and rightfully so. The United States is the fattest nation on the planet—a title I'm sure we'd prefer not to have, but one for which we are amply qualified. Our nation's obesity explosion is a complex problem with many culprits and players:

- Fast, nutritionally poor, high-calorie food that we can access 24/7
- Schools that are canceling physical education classes and organized physical activity
- A culture that is centered on static, seated activities for both work and play

Throw these together and you have a great recipe for Excessive Butt and Gut Epidemic Soup. But what it boils down to is that we move too little and eat too much.

However, there are hints of positive change within the food industry on the quality of products available, but they have a *long* way to go. And schools are becoming more aware of the importance of providing healthy meals to children and regular physical activities.

Although food quality may not be the "smoking gun" in the obesity epidemic, it is great place for you to start taking personal responsibility. You, and only you, can decide if you will fill your tank with "premium" nutrition. Only you can make the changes necessary to move about in a top-of-the-line piece of well-tuned machinery or fill up your tank with crap sure to keep you looking and feeling like a broken-down jalopy. Your food choices are fundamental to the success you have with your health and fitness. The simple fact is you are indeed what you eat, so choose carefully.

"Tell me what you eat,
and I will tell you what you are."

—JEAN-ANTHELME BRILLAT-SAVARIN (1755–1826)

It's Not Simply About Eating Less

You don't necessarily get in shape or improve your fitness by eating less. It's not about less—it's about better. A bagel and a chicken breast may be similar in total size, but I assure you that they have different nutritional values for your body. To get healthy, you have to learn what to eat and why. You have to learn why the bagel is the wrong choice and the chicken breast is the right one. The quantity and quality of the life you live depends on it.

Eating less may sound like a simple means of dealing with your weight problem and the truth is that it will give you fast results. That's exactly the problem. Individuals drastically cut their calories and quickly drop a bunch of weight. They may feel good for a while, because it's exciting to drop five to ten pounds in a couple of weeks. Quick short-term success will initially keep them going, and they may even cut calories further in a futile effort to have even more weight-loss success. However, as most of you know from real world experience, it's a plan that cannot be maintained. It's riddled with holes.

By taking in fewer calories, you immediately place your body in physiological shock. Instead of speeding up your metabolism (which is what you should be trying to do), you end of sending your body into a panic, forcing it to slow down. Your body is wired to survive and when you deal it a sudden severe drop in calories, it almost immediately becomes defensive. In these times of low calorie consumption, your body may actually cannibalize itself. Your body may choose to use muscle as a food and energy source rather than fat. Does anybody start a diet intending to *not* lose fat? Of course not.

Crash dieting results in the loss of your most valuable ally for weight reduction—your muscle. Without it, your metabolism shrinks and slows to a snail's pace. Here's the scenario: you lose twenty or thirty pounds, perhaps more, with a diet of low calorie and nutritionally poor food, and you couple this with no weight training. The result is a smaller version of your old self, with a lot less muscle and a slower metabolism. You are now a prime candidate for massive weight gains because you've made yourself an excellent machine for fat storage. I doubt if that was your goal. Welcome to the vicious cycle of yo-yo dieting.

The Bagel vs. the Chicken Breast

Remember the bagel and chicken breast? The typical large plain bagel has 360 calories and contains 2.4 grams of fat, 73 grams of refined carbohydrates, and 13.8 grams of incomplete protein. It's as crappy a nutritional ratio as you could imagine and I haven't even added any butter, cream cheese spread, or peanut butter. Those extra ingredients only make it uglier nutritionally. If you were pushing a plow daily for eight hours instead of pushing a pencil, the bagel might not be as much of an issue. But since 99 percent of us no longer bust sod for a living, it's a surefire combination to send us straight to fat city.

The principal problem with the bagel is the refined carbohydrates and lack of any real nutrition. Do you remember your kindergarten art projects? If you ran out of glue, you could just mix white flour with water and you had more glue. Well, you basically make a bagel, loaf of white bread, or cake the same way. Think about that when you reach for processed flour products next time. And how long do you think a plain bagel will keep you satisfied before you reach for more calories? Unless your body's burning 'em (calories), it's probably storing 'em as fat. Not what you want.

It's not that carbohydrates are a terrible food source—they just don't fit our times. The ancient Egyptians built the great pyramids on a diet consisting chiefly of grains, and specifically bread. Think they were fat? Fat chance. Moving fifty-ton stones in the African heat for ten hours a day has a way of working off those calories. Chances are that the bread they were eating wasn't refined and nutritionally empty, but rather stone-ground, whole-grain bread.

A grilled, six-ounce chicken breast has 284 calories, 76 calories less than a bagel. The chicken breast's calories are comprised of 8 grams of fat, no carbohydrates, and 53.4 grams of protein. Yes, the chicken breast has more fat, but it's a mere 6 grams, which will help give you a sense of satisfaction and fullness. A chicken breast is empty of carbohydrates and packed full of *the* nutrient that acts as the "building block" for every single cell in your body—protein.

*"Change your thoughts
and you change your world."*
—NORMAN VINCENT PEALE (1898–1993)

Don't Eat Five Meals a Day

I know, you've heard that the most effective way to consume your daily calories is in small, multiple meals, about every two to three hours, right? Fitness "experts" have argued and made a substantial case for the benefits of such an eating pattern, and they're not wrong—eating multiple meals throughout the day does have *real* benefits. I don't question the validity of the claim, but I do question when it should be implemented.

In a perfect world, I'd definitely advise people to eat moderately sized, balanced meals every three hours. Eating small, frequent meals has numerous benefits, such as stimulating your metabolism, curbing your appetite, and stabilizing your endocrine system (the release of insulin and other hormones), to name a few. However, I'm trying to ease you into a lifestyle change and putting too much on your platter, literally, is often a recipe for failure and frustration. Eating five to six small meals a day may have your plate overflowing.

I've seen it a thousand times—well-intentioned, seemingly motivated individuals decide to change their lives and this new "life" routine is so overwhelming, so consuming, that after a few weeks or maybe a month, they stop. It's too much too soon, like starting a running program with the Boston Marathon! I love enthusiasm, but too often we fall prey to this scenario because we're spoiled. We live in an instant gratification society, where we get what we want, when we want it. Though this might work when shopping on eBay, your health and fitness are a different animal.

Often, when we decide that it's finally time to get in shape, we often take a "no holds barred" approach. We immediately start a daily routine of running and weightlifting, visiting the gym every night. We make a run to the local health food store for the latest nutrition bars and supplements. We give our kitchen a makeover and restock it with what we believe are the right food choices. We buy new workout wardrobes, shoes, a lifting belt, and the latest exercise gloves.

While this all sounds well and good, the next morning's reality is inescapable. You awake clutching the pillow as if it's a life preserver, your body contoured around the pillow, cramped in a fetal position. You can barely pull yourself up from the bed. Once in the bathroom, you forgo actually brushing your hair because your shoulders, upper back, and chest are too sore. The hair brush might as well be an anvil. You do no better with brushing your teeth. Getting fully dressed takes a solid hour and once you've finally limped your way to the kitchen, you realize you're already late for work. The thought of egg whites makes you nauseous and, besides, the refrigerator is almost five feet away and you can't risk the trip. If you stumble and fall, you may not be able to get back on your feet. So, you grab the remaining cold coffee from last night's convenience store stop and make your way to the car. Welcome to day two!

Okay, I may be making the scenario a little dramatic, but I think you understand the point. And I'm sure the above story line is not without its sympathizers. Some of you are laughing and silently crying, knowing that you've been there to some degree and have a similar story. Let's not go there again.

Remember the story of the tortoise and the hare? Slow, steady, well-thought-out changes over time are the way to win this race. So, instead of just jumping feet first into the fire and thinking you need to eat five or six meals a day to be successful with your health and fitness goals, stop and ask yourself, how many *good* meals are you currently consuming a day? Are you getting a healthy balanced breakfast? What about lunch and dinner? Do your daily meals include a lean protein, plenty of green, leafy vegetables, and a small serving of a complex carbohydrate? Probably not.

Before you begin adding *more* meals to your daily diet, doesn't it make sense that you should establish three, balanced meals first? Start by eating three basic, healthy meals a day. When you are consistent in your workouts, your sleep, and eating healthy with your three basic meals, only then may it be appropriate to start adding additional small meals.

> *"The path to our destination is not always a straight one.*
> *We go down the wrong road, we get lost, we turn back.*
> *Maybe it doesn't matter which road we embark on.*
> *Maybe what matters is that we embark."*
>
> —BARBARA HALL

Stair-Stepping Your Weight Down

Let's keep it simple. Choose your food with the following guidelines in mind. First, lean protein is your new best friend: it's low in calories and slow to digest (which keeps you feeling full longer). Two, don't eat anything fried. Did I have to say that? Third, eat vegetables, which are low in calories and high in nutrition, which means you, can eat them all-day long. However, avoid vegetables smothered in butter or rich sauces. Steamed or raw vegetables with a little, low-calorie dressing (if needed) are perfect. Fourth, eat breakfast. Yes, it *is* the most important meal of the day. Get up and get used to it.

I am not a fan of calorie counting, but to some degree it is necessary. At least in the beginning, you need to get a grasp and a basic understanding of the calories in the foods you're eating. It's tedious and a pain in the ass, but it's also the only way you'll learn to eat healthy. And learning is the *real* key—your success in both establishing and preserving an improved state of health and fitness will largely be dependent on the knowledge you learn and then apply.

You can get sophisticated in deciding the exact amount of daily calories you should be consuming, but most of us do not need to get too complicated with calculating our total, daily caloric intake. For most of us, rough estimations are more than enough. Keep it simple! This book and this approach are designed mostly for those who are sedentary, individuals whose jobs and lives mainly involve sitting at a desk and pushing a pencil much of the day. And just for clarification, pushing a pencil or keypad does not qualify as resistance training.

The following five categories are meant to provide you with a *loose* guideline on how many total daily calories you should be consuming. To determine your calories, find your current body weight within one of the five categories. Then, using the recommending daily eating guideline, begin stair-stepping your weight down. Once you reach, or come within five pounds or so of, the lightest weight showed within the category, simply continue to the next category.

Don't skip categories! This is important. You're impatient, I know, everybody is. You've spent ten, twenty, thirty, or more years putting on those extra pounds and now you want it off in sixty days! That's normal, but it's not practical. This process will take time.

The suggested eating plans within the five categories are not set it stone. There may be a food I've selected that you either just plain hate or maybe you're allergic to it. So, you may need to adjust and substitute foods, but do so with the total calorie count in mind. It's not *all* about the calories, but it's essential that you not overlook or underestimate any calories you may unintentionally add to your daily eating. For instance; a glass of red wine at night seems harmless, but it's roughly 150 extra calories to your day's total. It adds up! Weight gain is a "snowball" effect—it builds slowly over time, creeping up on you. You may think that the little things (a bite of desert, a piece of bread, a few chips or cream in you coffee) won't matter, but they do. Soon those "little things" are happening with every meal and what was once 150 more calories becomes 500! Don't let little things creep into your diet.

You'll notice there are two items glaringly missing from this book and my approach—recipes and food lists. These two items are often used as nothing more than "filler" in most weight loss books, and I am not going to overwhelm you with endless, unnecessary recipes that you don't need and won't use. Nor am I going to provide you lists of "good" and "bad" foods. Why not? Because I think you know (in general) what makes up a "good" food and what makes up a "bad" food. Perhaps you've been lazy in your food choices up till now, but just use your common sense. More often that not, it's right, so trust it.

Remember, total calories are only a small part of long-term weight loss. The real key to success is choosing the best foods to make up those calories. *All calories are not created equal.* I've given you examples below of some positive choices. Healthy eating is about increasing the value of the foods you select.

LADIES AND GENTLEMEN, START YOUR ENGINES

Your Weight: 250 to 350 pounds

Your Total Daily Calories: 1,950 to 2,100

Your Meal Plan:

Breakfast—two eggs any style, two slices whole-wheat toast with
  sugar-free jam, and half a banana (500 calories)

Morning Snack—low-sugar yogurt with half a serving of whey
  protein powder (150 calories)

Lunch—Asian grilled chicken salad (300 calories)

Afternoon Snack—one apple and one cup of low-fat cottage cheese
  (290 calories)

Dinner—one grilled, seasoned chicken breast, one palm-size serving
  of steamed green beans or broccoli, and one cup of brown rice
  (510 calories)

Evening Snack—half a cup of edamame soybeans (200 calories)

You have to start somewhere. Recognizing that your weight has
reached this first category is sobering and depressing. It's a dose of reality we'd all like to avoid, but burying your head in the sand won't make it
go away. Take a good long look in the mirror. Is this how you want too
look and how you want to feel? If not, then do something about it. Not
next month or next week or even tomorrow—start today by making up
your mind that you want more out of life.

ROOM TO MOVE

Your Weight: 200 to 249 pounds

Your Total Daily Calories: 1,700 to 1,850

Your Meal Plan:

Breakfast—two high-protein breakfast bars (280 calories)

Snack—one serving of EAS Myoplex Light (190 calories)

Lunch—chicken burrito with beans, rice, and salsa (410 calories)

Snack—one cup of low-fat cottage cheese (200 calories)

Dinner—one grilled, seasoned chicken breast, one palm-size serving of steamed green beans or broccoli, and one medium baked potato (520 calories)

Snack—half a cup of edamame soybeans (200 calories)

I am not a fan of "cheat" days, although I know there are some diet programs that advise taking a day off from eating healthy. If you ask me, you've had plenty of cheat days—many of us have had thirty plus years of cheat days. By my calculations, that's 10,950 days of eating whatever you wished. That should have been plenty. No more cheat days and no more sabotaging your health. It's time to pay the piper.

SLIP SLIDING AWAY

Your Weight: 180 to 199 pounds

Your Total Daily Calories: 1,550 to 1,650

Your Meal Plan:

Breakfast—three egg whites, any style, half a cup of plain oatmeal with Splenda (200 calories)

Snack— half a cup of almonds (415 calories)

Lunch—Mandarin chicken salad (170 calories)

Snack—Met-Rx Meal Replacement Shake RTD 51 (240 calories)

Dinner—one grilled pork chop, one palm-size serving of steamed green beans or broccoli, and one palm-size serving of brown rice (410 calories)

Snack—low-fat yogurt (190 calories)

I can't tell you how long it will take you to move from one category to the next. Many factors have an influence on your weight: genetics, age, gender, exercise level, and, of course, resolve all play a role. I know you'd like to have a definitive "map" for your course, but it simply doesn't exist. There is no magic or luck involved. The dedication, discipline, and consistency you apply will determine your success. I am providing you direction and a destination, but the course you take is up to you.

CAN'T YOU ALMOST TASTE IT?

Your Weight: 150 to 179 pounds

Your Total Daily Calories: 1,350 to 1,500

Your Meal Plan:

Breakfast—English muffin with egg (290 calories)

Snack—EAS Myoplex Light, one serving (190 calories)

Lunch—turkey breast sandwich (280 calories)

Snack—half a cup of non-fat cottage cheese (60 calories)

Dinner—one grilled, seasoned chicken breast, one palm-size serving of steamed green beans or broccoli, and one small baked potato (420 calories)

Snack—half a cup of edamame soybeans (160 calories)

The fact is that the more weight you lose, the harder it is to lose weight. That's why when you begin changing your eating habits, you're more than likely to experience the greatest amount of weight loss in the least amount of time. That's the hook that the weight loss industry uses—that's how they're able to "pull the wool" over the consumer's eyes (*your* eyes) and keep you buying a product that has only short-term results. Consistency is the true key—changing your lifestyle for good and sticking with the program.

SHAZAM!

Your Weight: 120 to 149 pounds

Your Total Daily Calories: 1,200 to 1,300

Your Meal Plan:

Breakfast—four egg whites, any style, with a palm-size serving of broccoli (130 calories)

Snack—EAS Myoplex Light, one serving (190 calories)

Lunch—two slices of thin-crust cheese pizza (380 calories)

Snack—one small apple (80 calories)

Dinner—one grilled, seasoned chicken breast, one palm-size serving of steamed green beans or broccoli (200 calories)

Snack—one cup of edamame soybeans (250 calories)

Don't give me the "I want to enjoy life" excuse for your terrible eating decisions and behaviors. Quit feeding yourself that bull and cowboy up! If Burger King and Taco Bell are defining the joy of your existence, you've got more problems than this book can solve. Eat right, eat healthy, and start enjoying the *real* rewards of life. The values and experience garnered from living a balanced and healthy lifestyle are immeasurable. Start your investment now and reap the rewards!

"Good habits result from resisting temptation"

—ANCIENT PROVERB

Practice Consistency

I know what many of you are saying as you read through the eating out-lines I've provided: "I can't eat the same foods every day. That's boring." In my twenty plus years of personal training, one of the most common complaints (it's an excuse, let's call it what it is) I've heard from clients is "It's boring to eat healthy." Oh, if I only had a dollar for every time I've heard that. Well, here's what I know and you don't—your diet doesn't consist of much variety anyway. In fact, you eat damn near the same every day and I can prove it.

I start every new client with one simple exercise: I have them phy-sically record (with paper and pencil) *everything* they eat for 5–7 days. Then, we sit down and look at the nutritional composition of their diet. Typically, it's not very pretty. Most diets consist of way too many simple sugars (pop, candy, snacks, etc.) and many excessively processed carbohy-drates, such as white breads, pastas, and fried foods. But what is also glar-ingly obvious is how little variety is visible in most people's daily diet.

Breakfast is at the same drive-through every morning with the same menu selection (if breakfast is eaten at all). Lunch is almost always with co-workers at the same sandwich shop. The mid-afternoon snack is from the same hallway vending machine, and evening dinner is typically take-out from the same one or two restaurants. So, lack of variety of the diet isn't the problem. The problem is taste, or at least that's what you think. But taste isn't the problem either. The real problem is conditioning—emotional, social, and physical conditioning. Your poor eating behaviors are habits and the only way to change habits is to practice consistency; that is, consistency of new habits. Think it will be easy? Wrong, it'll be hard as hell. That's the nature of the beast. You have two choices: slay the beast or be a slave to it. You'll have to choose which you want.

"The body is an instrument, the mind its function,
the witness and reward of its operation."

—George Santayana

Quit Setting Goals!

If nothing I've said so far has caught you by surprise, the title of this section surely did. After all, we're a goal-driven society, reaching and straining for the elusive "carrot" in whatever form it may take. Whether it's climbing the corporate ladder, planning your retirement, or buying that next bigger and better house, we all have things we want. These elusive "things" become our goals, and the achievement of these goals then becomes the means by which we measure our lives. Their achievement ties closely to our very sense of "self"; in fact, they're almost interwoven.

Goals can be powerful motivators, but too often goals become hapless traps, unattainable ideals that are out of our reach and beyond our scope of accomplishment. Why? Because goals left unchecked can become a destructive focus and leave us blind to the real mechanisms necessary for success. These mechanisms are what I like to call "turning the wheel." Turning the wheel is how you'll accomplish your goals—the mundane, daily rigor of regular exercise and better eating choices that will eventually lead you to your physical goals. They're neither exciting, "sexy," nor glamorous. They are what they are, the necessary cogs whose revolution ensures success. Your goal is to continue "turning your wheel," day in and day out.

How much would you like to weigh—160 pounds? 140 pounds? Maybe even 120 pounds? Its accomplishment is tethered to your wheel like an umbilical cord. Your ultimate success will depend on your ability to turn your wheel. Without it, your goal is just a wish. And as my Uncle Jim is so fond of saying, "Wish in one hand and shit in the other. See which one piles up first."

Chapter 3

THE BUTT AND GUT PROGRAM

"Dwell not upon thy weariness, thy strength shall be according to the measure of thy desire."

—ARAB PROVERB

Targeted Training Done Wisely

You store a larger percentage of excess body weight on your stomach and hips. The Butt & Gut Program focuses on those two areas of the body. Male and female physiques store excess body weight in the same manner, but they divide that storage in different areas—the butt in females, the gut in males. However, eat badly enough, for long enough, and stay on your ass more than you should, and eventually you'll get fat all over. But there's no denying that men develop "beer bellies" and women "saddlebags." Just look around. It's preprogrammed in our DNA. The question is, what can we do about it?

The Butt & Gut Program is not a "spot-reducing" program. You'll not be able to get away with exercising *only* your "trouble spots" forever, nor should you. There are over 600 muscles in the human body, and you'll eventually need to practice and incorporate balanced, healthy conditioning. Think of your body as a car. You need your car to run effectively and efficiently. You can ensure that by properly keeping the tires inflated, changing the oil, choosing the proper fuel, and regular maintenance. You cannot just change the oil or just put gas in. Doing so would be negligent. If you only care for one aspect of your car, eventually your car will break down. How is your body any different?

You want to get rid of your excess butt and gut, so out of the gate the Butt & Gut Program has a focus on those two areas of your body. This is the "hook," but it's a hook with a purpose. The purpose is to get you on the path: get you active, get you some results, get you up off your ass and exercising, and get you beginning to make better eating decisions. However, it's not smoke and mirrors. The Butt & Gut Program is effective. It'll work, but the question is, will you?

The Butt & Gut Program is a means to an end—a start, a step, the beginning of a new and exciting change in your life. It targets what a great many of us feel are our "trouble spots," but it's merely a crack in the door. You'll have to swing the door wider, open it up, because you'll never know what's behind it unless you push it all the way open. So, go ahead, give it a push. Push your door all the way open.

> *"Opportunity is missed by most people because it is dressed in overalls and looks like work."*
> —THOMAS A. EDISON (1847–1931)

120 Minutes, 120 Days, and the Sky's the Limit!

You will get out of Butt & Gut Program exactly what you put into it. It's not magic, easy, or quick. It's not a pill, a diet, or a drink. It's work. Twenty minutes, six days a week, for 120 days. Miss workouts and you miss opportunities. Every day you put "crap" in your mouth, or stay in bed instead of exercising, are days you fall behind. You could make them up, but why would you? Do it right the first time. What are you waiting for? Time marches on and either you seize it and wring it for all it's worth or you can sit on the sidelines and keep score. You *will* lose weight and get in better shape with the Butt & Gut Program, but *only* if you put in the time and effort.

The Butt & Gut Program lasts 120 days, but that's a bit misleading because it's essentially a *beginning* program, one that prepares you for a lifestyle of health and fitness. Yes, lifestyle—as in something you'll do the rest of your life. Daunting? Possibly. But remember, the value of exercise and healthy eating lies not in its completion, but in the voyage. You are now on a life voyage, a journey of continued success and invigorating challenges. It's a hell of a trip indeed.

Take a deep breath and swell with a little pride. You're about to do what most people won't do these days—*work*! You're taking the road least traveled, but in the end you'll be better for it: you'll walk with a little different gait and your head will be held a little higher. You'll present a package forged by dedication, discipline, and consistency, not some surgeon's knife. And when an acquaintance at a party leans over and whispers to you, "You look great. What 'work' did you have done?" you won't have to cover your mouth, glance around the room, and then casually whisper back, "I had liposuction." Instead, you're liable to stand on your chair, smile ear to ear, and shout across the room, "I've been busting my ass!"

> *"Few things are impossible to diligence and skill. Great works are performed not by strength, but perseverance."*
> —Samuel Johnson (1709–1784)

Getting Off the Throne

You must learn to squat correctly. It is a foundational movement that will provide you with the bedrock of your conditioning and it is a cornerstone movement of most of the lower body exercises in the Butt & Gut Program. Learning to squat correctly will improve your posture, your coordination, your balance, and your body awareness skills, not to mention the obvious effects on strength, power, and conditioning. However, it is neither easy to perform nor learn, because squatting is a challenging movement, both physically and mentally. That's both why everybody should learn to squat and nobody does. You will learn to squat!

The squat movement is akin to many the movements in the Butt & Gut Program, which includes multiple variations of squatting, such as the Sumo Squat, Jump Squats, Chair Squats, and various Supported Squats, to name a few. And the motion of the squat is also fundamental to the whole host of different lunge techniques you'll be performing with the Butt & Gut Program as well.

Why is the squat so important? Simple—when we talk about getting "bang for your buck," then there's no argument for any other exercise. They are roughly 600 muscles in the human body, and performing a full-range, body-weight squat uses about half of them. Now that's a return on your investment! This is also why when fitness professionals talk about the squat, they often refer to it as "The King": no other exercise even comes close to stressing the body to the same degree or magnitude.

Squatting makes your heart beat fast and your lungs burn; and just for clarity, that's good. This is also principally why, when you perform the Butt & Gut Program, you'll start with the gut exercise first. When you finish the leg portion of the program, your breathing will be labored enough to make training the gut difficult.

Here are five key points to remember when performing the various squats and lunges of the Butt & Gut Program:

Keep your head up, your shoulders back, and your upper back arched. This is much more difficult than it sounds but essential to properly performing the movements and heightening their role.

Preserve the position of your upper body over your hips. In the beginning, this is difficult because of your lack of lower body strength. You'll want to lean forward on many of the lower body movements. Doing so changes the distribution of your upper body weight and seemingly makes the exercise easier. Making the exercises easier is not our goal; strive instead to make them harder.

Learn to keep your gut muscles "tight" or semi-contracted during the lower body workout. This stabilizes your torso, allowing your legs to drive securely from beneath. Research has proven that simple, basic body-weight squats activate your midsection muscles to the same degree as many specific abdominal exercises.

During a squat, always press from and through your heels. This is one of the more difficult aspects of correctly squatting, but it will improve both your ankle and your hip flexibility. As you extend through the lower body movements, you may notice that most of your body weight is on the balls of your feet or even your toes. Work hard to correct this by keeping your body weight on your heels throughout the full range of the motion.

Your knees should always follow the direction of your toes. Whether it be a lunge variation or a squat, do not let your knees travel either outside or inside the line fixed by your heels and toes.

You *have* to be able to get up and down—it's fundamental to life. Whether you're twenty years old or eighty, getting up and down is a movement you do daily. Getting out of your work chair, off the floor from playing with your kids, or off the "throne" in the morning are movements akin to the squat. Keep your legs strong with the squat and you'll be able to perform all of the above with your pride and dignity intact.

Why Squat?

- Stimulates your metabolism
- Increased growth hormone production
- Improves your balance
- Strengthens your knees and hips
- Burns a lot of calories!

> *"A goal without a plan is just a wish."*
> —Antoine de Saint-Exupery (1900–1944)

Suck It In

How many times have you heard that phrase? For many of us, the secret to having a pleasing waistline has centered on our ability to pull our abdominals inward toward our spine. It's actually a movement known as the stomach vacuum and it isn't without value as a mid-section exercise. Sucking in your gut uses a deep abdominal muscle called the transverse abdominus that has been made famous by the "core" and Pilates trends. However, the stomach vacuum isn't necessarily a "foundational" movement of the mid-section the way the squat is to the lower body.

If you wish to target the outer layers of abdominal muscles, look no further than the basic crunch. Correctly performing the crunch movement is not difficult. It is a short, focused movement specifically targeting the rectus abdominus—your "six pack." Unlike the squat, however, the crunch's physical impact is targeted. Where the squat involves literally hundreds of muscles, in comparison the crunch involves relatively few. It is as close to what most people consider an "isolation" movement as is possible. However, all things considered, the crunch is still a "central" movement for the abdominal area and foundational to every other mid-section exercise.

Here are a few key points for ensuring that you perform the crunch correctly.

- Short, tight, and controlled. Repeat this endlessly to yourself as you perform the crunch.

- Don't necessarily think about coming 'up" when performing the crunch. Instead, think about shortening the distance between your sternum and your pelvis.

- Don't pull or nod your head. The first is bad for your neck and the second is likely to give it a good workout. I doubt you want either.

- Roll your head and shoulders slightly. Visualize pressing your belly button down and your lower back into the floor.

- There are a "ton" of crunch variations. Start simple and master the basics.

For complete and thorough mid-section conditioning, you'll need to incorporate a multitude of movements and exercises. Think of the crunch as one of those many "tools," one of many mid-section tools you'll eventually know, learn, and master. As you expand your knowledge of effective mid-section movements, keep in mind the simple mechanics of the basic crunch—those same mechanics will apply to the majority of abdominal exercises.

Why Crunch?

- It's simple and effective.
- It's exercise you can perform anytime and anywhere.
- Specifically targets your abdominal rectus, the abdominal muscles utilized on every mid-section movement.
- There's virtually no chance of lower back strain or injury.
- Some aspect of the crunch's mechanics is an integral part of every abdominal exercise.

> *"When you reach for the stars*
> *you may not quite get one,*
> *but you won't come up with*
> *a handful of mud either."*
>
> —LEO BURNETT

Stairway to Heaven

Running or walking stairs is a critical part of the Butt & Gut Program. The movement associated with either walking or running stairs is substantially superior, for many reasons, to running or walking on a flat surface. It also happens to be hard. That's why stairs are a part of this program and why you'll be doing them.

You're not going to be doing stairs simply because it's hard. It would also be hard to sleep on a bed of nails, but I haven't included that into the Butt & Gut Program. Yet. Stairs are hard because they're physically demanding: the mechanics of climbing stairs compared to traditional walking or running requires more motion, and thus more muscle involvement. The greater the motion and the more muscles used, the more calories burned—and that's the golden egg of exercise. Work hard but also work smarter. Driving a nail in your hand every day would hurt like hell, but it's not going to improve your fitness. Pain for pain's sake is not what we're after.

Climbing stairs is an effective exercise because each time you step, you place your foot up and slightly forward. To reach the next step level, the foot you've just placed must bear your weight and drive your body upward. To some degree, running stairs is resistance training. Unlike running or walking on a flat surface, where your body moves laterally along the plane of the ground, with stairs your legs must drive your body up and forward. The entire motion needs a much larger range of action from your knee and your hip. It's this increased range that results in more muscle recruitment and so more calories burned. It has the added benefit of also being low impact by significantly reducing the pounding your knees and hips take from walking or (especially) running.

I am not a fan of traditional running or walking. As part of a balanced fitness program, they either provide incomplete conditioning or simply come at too high an expense in terms of potential injuries. Both forms of exercise are popular because they're simple—no need for equipment or gym membership. While that may sound like an attractive form of exercise, you can do better. Do it with stairs: exercising on stairs also needs no equipment, no experience, and no gym membership; oh, and *stairs work!*

Here are a few things to keep in mind while doing stairs.

Run up but walk down. Running up stairs is relatively easy on your joints. Running down them is as equally hard on them.

Pump your arms with your legs. Keep your elbow slightly bent but secured in place. Your elbow should swing an equal distance from front to back of your mid-line.

Focus on landing lightly with each step. Try to place your body weight equally across the entire foot.

Drive your body explosively up with each step.

Keep your shoulders back and your chest up ensuring good posture.

Why Stairs?

- Increased range of motion
- Less potentially damaging impact
- Increased muscle action
- Burns more calories than traditional running or walking
- Strengthens your knees and hips

> *"To follow, without halt, one aim:*
> *there's the secret of success."*
>
> —ANNA PAVLOVA (1885–1931)

Priming the Pump

Warming up is the easy part but it's a part nonetheless, and one you shouldn't ignore. Warming up shouldn't require more than 3–5 minutes of your total exercise time, so get up, get going, and get it done. The simplest and easiest means of warming up is simply to walk in place. Just stand in place and begin performing a soldier's march. Start slow, building both your speed and the height of your legs' motion. Apply the same crescendo-type approach of movement to your arms as well: slowly pump them in the beginning and incrementally increase your arm speed and total range of motion, mirroring your lower body. Within about two minutes, you should be hitting a good pace. Keep that intensity for a few more minutes. Catch your breath, then get to the Butt & Gut workout.

Warming Up

- Start slow and build the intensity.
- Simply walk in place and pump your arms.
- Jumping rope is also a simple and effective warm up.
- Warm up for a total time of 3–5 minutes.

*"If you limit your choices only to what seems possible
or reasonable, you disconnect yourself from what you
truly want, and all that is left is a compromise."*

—ROBERT FRITZ

The Complete Butt & Gut Workout

The Butt & Gut Program is unique in that it's an exercise program that needs no weights, no dumbbells, no bench, no exercise balls, no Ab-roller, no bike, and no treadmill. You need nothing for this program but a pulse and an attitude. This program uses you and you alone as both the instrument of exercise and the means of self-torture.

There are two parts to each thirty-day segment of the Butt & Gut Program, body-weight exercises (movements that use your own weight for resistance) and cardiovascular conditioning. Both are equally valuable and each plays a distinct role. Three days a week you'll perform three body-weight movements for your butt and three body-weight movements for your gut. Though these exercises specifically target your butt and gut, they have the added benefit of working a whole host of other muscles as well.

Though you may think or have heard otherwise, muscles *do not* work in complete isolation. Even "isolation" exercises incorporate the use of other muscles. Sometimes these extra muscles are simply called into play to support or stabilize the primary muscle's motion, but they're involved nonetheless. Even though muscles by definition do not work alone, we can still group many exercises as isolation movements. The number of joints involved in a movement defines what most experts classify as "isolation" exercises—movements that engage one primary joint, such as a standard barbell curl, a movement primarily involving the elbow.

Isolation exercises have a role and can be a valuable part of an exercise routine. However,, the average individual should spend most their time exercising with movements that incorporate a myriad of muscles and multiple joints. It's the "bang for your buck" argument—more muscles worked means more calories burned. The Butt & Gut Program takes advantage of this idea.

On the Ascent

The Butt & Gut Program is what I call an "ascending" program, meaning that as you progress through the program, the intensity of the time spent exercising also increases. You'll do this by continually adding to the total number of exercise sets completed, adding to the total number of exercise repetitions, and increasing the intensity of exercise by selecting movements that have a higher degree of difficulty. I apply the same basic method to the cardiovascular part of the Butt & Gut Program. Every thirty days of the program, you'll incrementally increase the time you spend walking stairs. For instance, during the first thirty days, you'll perform a brisk fifteen-minute walk immediately followed by five minutes of walking stairs. By the last thirty days, you'll be walking stairs a full twenty minutes, three days a week.

The Butt & Gut Program is time efficient and simple to understand, but don't misinterpret those words to mean "quick" or "easy." You'll work hard with this program: you're going to sweat and you're going be sore.

You can complete the Butt & Gut Program anywhere, which is the distinct advantage of the exercises in the program. You can do the Butt & Gut Program on the road, on vacation, in your office, in your bedroom, or on the beach. Forget about a gym membership, fighting traffic while driving across town to the club, and dealing with surly desk staff or underpaid and over-exercised instructors. Your new gym is always open and ready. Even better, if you don't like the results, you know exactly who to blame! So, start busting your butt and gut!

The Butt & Gut Program at a Glance

- Six 20-minute workouts a week
  - Three cardiovascular workouts
  - Three resistance workouts
- No equipment necessary
- Three butt exercises
- Three gut exercises
- Stairs!

"A positive attitude may not solve all your problems,
but it will annoy enough people to make it worth the effort."
—HERM ALBRIGHT (1876–1944)

The First Thirty (Weeks One to Four)

During the first thirty days of the Butt & Gut Program, you'll learn and perform six gut exercises—three exercises during the first two weeks and three different exercises during the last two weeks. You'll also be learning six butt exercises. Always perform the gut exercises before the butt exercises, which ensures that your breathing (which may be heavy after completing the butt exercises) doesn't interfere with properly controlling and contracting your gut muscles.

You'll perform two sets of ten repetitions (2 x 10) with each exercise during the first two weeks (fourteen days) of this program. Then, during the next two weeks, you will increase the total sets but not the number of repetitions—you'll perform three sets of ten repetitions (3 x 10) with each exercise.

I have set the recovery (resting) time between each set at a vigorous twenty seconds. This ensures a quick pace of exercise and has the added benefit of being stimulating to your cardiovascular system. Also, you should finish each workout within a maximum of twenty minutes. If you rest longer than twenty seconds, you won't complete the Butt & Gut Program within twenty minutes, which is your goal each time you exercise.

The First Thirty Days

- Two sets of ten repetitions (2 x 10) with each exercise the first two weeks
- Three sets of ten repetitions (3 x 10) with each exercise the next two weeks
- Do your gut exercises before your butt exercises
- Rest *only* twenty seconds between sets
- Complete each workout within twenty minutes
- Pay close attention to your form

Variety is a key element to sticking with an exercise program, which is why every two weeks of this sixteen-week program you'll be expanding your exercise knowledge base with three new gut exercises and three new butt exercises. Don't just *do* the exercises, learn them and increase your personal "bank" of exercises. The more you learn, the longer you'll last. It is important that you perform these movements correctly, so pay close attention to both the exercise descriptions and the accompanying photographs. Doing so increases their effectiveness and reduces the unlikely chance of injury.

Week One

This is as easy as it gets and it's that way for a reason. Many of you will feel as though these first couple of weeks of workouts are unchallenging. But you've got to start somewhere and starting somewhere begins with a consistent pattern of regular exercise. I'm concerned with having you establish a habit of exercising. You may be able to exercise longer and with greater intensity, but the question is, can you keep on doing it?

See Chapters 4 and 5 for detailed instructions (with accompanying photos) on how to properly perform each exercise. There are also additional exercise for your butt and gut to help vary your routine.

DAY	EXERCISE	DURATION/ SETS & REPS
Day One	Brisk Walk	20 minutes
Day Two	Basic Crunch	2 x 10
	Frog Crunch	2 x 10
	Single-Leg Raise	2 x 10
	Chair Squats with Pause	2 x 10
	Butt-Ups	2 x 10
	Chest on Floor Single-Leg Raise	2 x 10
Day Three	Brisk Walk	20 minutes
Day Four	Basic Crunch	2 x 10
	Frog Crunch	2 x 10
	Single-Leg Raise	2 x 10
	Chair Squats with Pause	2 x 10
	Butt-Ups	2 x 10
	Chest on Floor Single-Leg Raise	2 x 10
Day Five	Brisk Walk	20 minutes
Day Six	Basic Crunch	2 x 10
	Frog Crunch	2 x 10
	Single-Leg Raise	2 x 10
	Chair Squats with Pause	2 x 10
	Butt-Ups	2 x 10
	Chest on Floor Single-Leg Raise	2 x 10

Week Two

These first few weeks of the Butt & Gut Program are small steps toward much larger ones you'll be taking as the program progresses. I know you're in a hurry, but this journey has no shortcuts—they don't exist. You simply must incorporate regular exercise into your daily life. Some of you may be starting over; for many, you're just starting out. Either way, the rules are the same: take your time, be consistent, and establish the habit of exercise.

DAY	EXERCISE	DURATION/ SETS & REPS
Day One	Brisk Walk	20 minutes
Day Two	Basic Crunch	2 x 10
	Frog Crunch	2 x 10
	Single-Leg Raise	2 x 10
	Chair Squats with Pause	2 x 10
	Butt-Ups	2 x 10
	Chest on Floor Single-Leg Raise	2 x 10
Day Three	Brisk Walk	20 minutes
Day Four	Basic Crunch	2 x 10
	Frog Crunch	2 x 10
	Single-Leg Raise	2 x 10
	Chair Squats with Pause	2 x 10
	Butt-Ups	2 x 10
	Chest on Floor Single-Leg Raise	2 x 10
Day Five	Brisk Walk	20 minutes
Day Six	Basic Crunch	2 x 10
	Frog Crunch	2 x 10
	Single-Leg Raise	2 x 10
	Chair Squats with Pause	2 x 10
	Butt-Ups	2 x 10
	Chest on Floor Single-Leg Raise	2 x 10

Week Three

Each week will be tough. There will be days, weeks, even months when you don't want to be exercising. That's true of everybody. Don't believe the day is coming when you'll spring from your bed with a smile and walk stairs for the sheer fun of it. That's BS, and anybody who tells you otherwise is also selling you something you don't need, won't use, or both.

DAY	EXERCISE	DURATION/ SETS & REPS
Day One	Brisk Walk	15 minutes
	Stairs	5 minutes
Day Two	Basic Crunch	3 x 10
	Cross-Body Crunch	3 x 10
	Hip Lifts	3 x 10
	Chair Squats	3 x 10
	Assisted Stationary Lunge with Range Limit	3 x 10
	Bent-Knee Donkey Kick	3 x 10
Day Three	Brisk Walk	15 minutes
	Stairs	5 minutes
Day Four	Basic Crunch	3 x 10
	Cross-Body Crunch	3 x 10
	Hip Lifts	3 x 10
	Chair Squats	3 x 10
	Assisted Stationary Lunge with Range Limit	3 x 10
	Bent-Knee Donkey Kick	3 x 10
Day Five	Brisk Walk	15 minutes
	Stairs	5 minutes
Day Six	Basic Crunch	3 x 10
	Cross Body Crunch	3 x 10
	Hip Lifts	3 x 10
	Chair Squats	3 x 10
	Assisted Stationary Lunge with Range Limit	3 x 10
	Bent-Knee Donkey Kick	3 x 10

Week Four

Congratulations! Depending on how disciplined you've been with both your eating behaviors and your exercise, you may already be experiencing some noticeable changes. And regardless of whether you can see any differences or not, for sure you feel better. You're doing something positive and you're taking control. Yes, exercise is physical, but it's also psychological.

DAY	EXERCISE	DURATION/ SETS & REPS
Day One	Brisk Walk	15 minutes
	Stairs	5 minutes
Day Two	Basic Crunch	3 x 10
	Cross-Body Crunch	3 x 10
	Hip Lifts	3 x 10
	Chair Squats	3 x 10
	Assisted Stationary Lunge with Range Limit	3 x 10
	Bent-Knee Donkey Kick	3 x 10
Day Three	Brisk Walk	15 minutes
	Stairs	5 minutes
Day Four	Basic Crunch	3 x 10
	Cross-Body Crunch	3 x 10
	Hip Lifts	3 x 10
	Chair Squats	3 x 10
	Assisted Stationary Lunge with Range Limit	3 x 10
	Bent-Knee Donkey Kick	3 x 10
Day Five	Brisk Walk	15 minutes
	Stairs	5 minutes
Day Six	Basic Crunch	3 x 10
	Cross-Body Crunch	3 x 10
	Hip Lifts	3 x 10
	Chair Squats	3 x 10
	Assisted Stationary Lunge with Range Limit	3 x 10
	Bent-Knee Donkey Kick	3 x 10

"It seems to me that people have a vast potential. Most people can do extraordinary things if they have the confidence or take the risks. Yet most people don't. They sit in front of the telly and treat life as if it goes on forever."

—Philip Adams

The Second Thirty (Weeks Five to Eight)

The "nuts and bolts" of this program remain almost the same during the second month—what changes is the intensity. I increase the intensity with several mechanisms. One means is an increase in total repetitions: during the Second Thirty, you'll be increasing your repetitions with each set by five. By increasing the total repetitions from ten to fifteen, we measurably increase the exercise workload. In plain language, that means the set will be more difficult. I've also selected exercises that are more difficult to perform. This increase in difficulty results in yet another increase in the overall intensity of your exercise.

Finally, I've also increased your total "stairs" time. Starting now, you'll complete ten minutes of stairs during the first half of the Second Thirty and fifteen minutes for the last half. As you're probably finding out, running stairs is hard. That's why it's part of this program and that's why you're doing it! Don't overlook the role that running stairs plays in this program, in your conditioning, and in your success. Stairs work!

The Second Thirty Days

- Increase your repetitions for each set to fifteen
- Increase your total stairs time during the weeks five and six from five minutes to ten minutes
- Rest *only* twenty seconds between sets
- Complete each workout within twenty minutes
- Increase your total stairs time to fifteen minutes during weeks seven and eight

Week Five

It will be easy to quit at any time during the Butt & Gut Program. That's both the problem and lure of quitting—it's easy. Remember that, because as this program progresses, you must constantly choose the harder path, the path that will test your mettle. If you want the carrot, you're going to have to plant the seed, pull the weeds, hoe the garden, and harvest the crop.

DAY	EXERCISE	DURATION/ SETS & REPS
Day One	Brisk Walk	10 minutes
	Stairs	10 minutes
Day Two	Legs Straight and Crossed Crunch	3 x 15
	Figure Four Cross-Body Crunch	3 x 15
	Hip Rolls	3 x 15
	Sumo Stance Chair Squat	3 x 15
	Feet Forward Squats	3 x 15
	Heel in Chair Butt-Ups	3 x 15
Day Three	Brisk Walk	10 minutes
	Stairs	10 minutes
Day Four	Legs Straight and Crossed Crunch	3 x 15
	Figure Four Cross-Body Crunch	3 x 15
	Hip Rolls	3 x 15
	Sumo Stance Chair Squat	3 x 15
	Feet Forward Squats	3 x 15
	Heel in Chair Butt-Ups	3 x 15
Day Five	Brisk Walk	10 minutes
	Stairs	10 minutes
Day Six	Legs Straight and Crossed Crunch	3 x 15
	Figure Four Cross-Body Crunch	3 x 15
	Hip Rolls	3 x 15
	Sumo Stance Chair Squat	3 x 15
	Feet Forward Squats	3 x 15
	Heel in Chair Butt-Ups	3 x 15

Week Six

It's all about choices—choosing to exercise instead of sleeping that extra thirty minutes in the morning, choosing to walk a couple floors of stairs instead of riding in the elevator, choosing to eat something healthy. What we get out of life is what we choose. If you don't like what you've chosen, you know who to blame.

DAY	EXERCISE	DURATION/ SETS & REPS
Day One	Brisk Walk	10 minutes
	Stairs	10 minutes
Day Two	Legs Straight and Crossed Crunch	3 x 15
	Figure Four Cross-Body Crunch	3 x 15
	Hip Rolls	3 x 15
	Sumo Stance Chair Squat	3 x 15
	Feet Forward Squats	3 x 15
	Heel in Chair Butt-Ups	3 x 15
Day Three	Brisk Walk	10 minutes
	Stairs	10 minutes
Day Four	Legs Straight and Crossed Crunch	3 x 15
	Figure Four Cross-Body Crunch	3 x 15
	Hip Rolls	3 x 15
	Sumo Stance Chair Squat	3 x 15
	Feet Forward Squats	3 x 15
	Heel in Chair Butt-Ups	3 x 15
Day Five	Brisk Walk	10 minutes
	Stairs	10 minutes
Day Six	Legs Straight and Crossed Crunch	3 x 15
	Figure Four Cross-Body Crunch	3 x 15
	Hip Rolls	3 x 15
	Sumo Stance Chair Squats	3 x 15
	Feet Forward Squats	3 x 15
	Heel in Chair Butt-Ups	3 x 15

Week Seven

You may have to walk this path alone. You will not find crowds on the paths forged by individuals making hard, difficult choices. The path least traveled is not the one with a line. Know that from the start you can't rely on or expect help from anyone. Help may come, but if it does consider it a bonus not a constant source of aid. Even with Tonto, he was still the Lone Ranger.

DAY	EXERCISE	DURATION/ SETS & REPS
Day One	Brisk Walk	5 minutes
	Stairs	15 minutes
Day Two	Hip Rolls with Lift	3 x 15
	Feet Up, Ankles Crossed Crunch	3 x 15
	Body Plank	3 x 15
	Assisted Stationary Lunges	3 x 15
	Straight-Leg Rear Raise	3 x 15
	Sumo Butt-Ups with Pause	3 x 15
Day Three	Brisk Walk	5 minutes
	Stairs	15 minutes
Day Four	Hip Rolls with Lift	3 x 15
	Feet Up, Ankles Crossed Crunch	3 x 15
	Body Plank	3 x 15
	Assisted Stationary Lunges	3 x 15
	Straight-Leg Rear Raise	3 x 15
Day Five	Brisk Walk	5 minutes
	Stairs	15 minutes
Day Six	Hip Rolls with Lift	3 x 15
	Feet Up, Ankles Crossed Crunch	3 x 15
	Body Plank	3 x 15
	Assisted Stationary Lunges	3 x 15
	Straight-Leg Rear Raises	3 x 15

Week Eight

Halfway there? Yes and no. I've structured the Butt & Gut Program over sixteen weeks, but as I've told you before, this is only the beginning. This is an introductory program to establishing a health and fitness lifestyle. You're halfway through the Butt & Gut Program. Take great pride in that. You're on your way, but quit looking for the finish line. You're crossing it every day.

DAY	EXERCISE	DURATION/ SETS & REPS
Day One	Brisk Walk	5 minutes
	Stairs	15 minutes
Day Two	Hip Rolls with Lift	3 x 15
	Feet Up, Ankles Crossed Crunch	3 x 15
	Body Plank	3 x 15
	Assisted Stationary Lunges	3 x 15
	Straight-Leg Rear Raise	3 x 15
	Sumo Butt-Ups with Pause	3 x 15
Day Three	Brisk Walk	5 minutes
	Stairs	15 minutes
Day Four	Hip Rolls with Lift	3 x 15
	Feet Up, Ankles Crossed Crunch	3 x 15
	Body Plank	3 x 15
	Assisted Stationary Lunges	3 x 15
	Straight-Leg Rear Raise	3 x 15
Day Five	Brisk Walk	5 minutes
	Stairs	15 minutes
Day Six	Hip Rolls with Lift	3 x 15
	Feet Up, Ankles Crossed Crunch	3 x 15
	Body Plank	3 x 15
	Assisted Stationary Lunges	3 x 15
	Straight-Leg Rear Raise	3 x 15

*"Having once decided to achieve a certain task,
achieve it at all costs of tedium and distaste.
The gain in self-confidence of having accomplished
a tiresome labor is immense."*

—ARNOLD BENNETT

The Third Thirty (Weeks Nine to Twelve)

The Third Thirty incorporates more subtle changes to the Butt & Gut Program. As before, the exercises have changed and you'll be learning new movements for both your butt and your gut. The repetitions for each exercise remain the same (fifteen), but I am increasing the total sets completed with each exercise from three to four. Remember, you still must keep your total rest time between sets to about twenty seconds.

For weeks nine and ten, your walk-to-stairs ratio remains the same: five minutes of brisk walking followed by fifteen minutes of stairs. However, beginning with week eleven, your total stairs time has now reached its peak, *twenty minutes*! From this point on, your cardio workouts are stairs and stairs only. It hurts so good.

The Third Thirty Days

- Four sets with each exercise
- Fifteen repetitions with each set
- Rest *only* twenty seconds between sets
- Complete each workout in twenty minutes
- Increase your total stairs time from fifteen to twenty minutes during weeks eleven and twelve

Week Nine

You have to focus every single day, every single week. Every day, remind yourself of your goals, your objectives, and why you're exercising. It will try your character and test your soul. Every day, you will have to make the hard choice to stick with it. Temptation is everywhere, but don't avoid it—look it square in the eye, stare it down, and walk right over it.

DAY	EXERCISE	DURATION/ SETS & REPS
Day One	Brisk Walk	5 minutes
	Stairs	15 minutes
Day Two	Leg Raises	4 x 15
	Arms Overhead Crunch	4 x 15
	Side Plank with Hip Raise	4 x 15
	Sumo Jump Squat to Soldier Stand	4 x 15
	Ski Lunge	4 x 15
	Side Leg Raise	4 x 15
Day Three	Brisk Walk	5 minutes
	Stairs	15 minutes
Day Four	Leg Raises	4 x 15
	Arms Overhead Crunch	4 x 15
	Side Plank with Hip Raise	4 x 15
	Sumo Jump Squat to Soldier Stand	4 x 15
	Ski Lunge	4 x 15
	Side Leg Raise	4 x 15
Day Five	Brisk Walk	5 minutes
	Stairs	15 minutes
Day Six	Leg Raises	4 x 15
	Arms Overhead Crunch	4 x 15
	Side Plank with Hip Raise	4 x 15
	Sumo Jump Squat to Soldier Stand	4 x 15
	Ski Lunge	4 x 15
	Side Leg Raise	4 x 15

Week Ten

This is a path you may walk alone, but that doesn't mean you can't try to cultivate followers. In fact, it's your duty. Share your success, don't horde it. Can you think of a better gift? Do you know anyone who doesn't want to be in better condition and have more self-confidence? Preach your cause at every opportunity.

DAY	EXERCISE	DURATION/ SETS & REPS
Day One	Brisk Walk	5 minutes
	Stairs	15 minutes
Day Two	Leg Raises	4 x 15
	Arms Overhead Crunch	4 x 15
	Side Plank with Hip Raise	4 x 15
	Sumo Jump Squat to Soldier Stand	4 x 15
	Ski Lunge	4 x 15
	Side Leg Raise	4 x 15
Day Three	Brisk Walk	5 minutes
	Stairs	15 minutes
Day Four	Leg Raises	4 x 15
	Arms Overhead Crunch	4 x 15
	Side Plank with Hip Raise	4 x 15
	Sumo Jump Squat to Soldier Stand	4 x 15
	Ski Lunge	4 x 15
	Side Leg Raise	4 x 15
Day Five	Brisk Walk	5 minutes
	Stairs	15 minutes
Day Six	Leg Raises	4 x 15
	Arms Overhead Crunch	4 x 15
	Side Plank with Hip Raise	4 x 15
	Sumo Jump Squat to Soldier Stand	4 x 15
	Ski Lunge	4 x 15
	Side Leg Raise	4 x 15

Week Eleven

I know what you're thinking, maybe even saying: "Exercising every day is so boring and monotonous." News bulletin, folks—that's life. Think about it. You go to the same job every day, take the same route, see the same people, and go through the same routine. For most of us, life is pretty predictable. Don't blame exercise—your life wasn't that exciting to begin with.

DAY	EXERCISE	DURATION/ SETS & REPS
Day One	Stairs	20 minutes
Day Two	Pilates 100	1 x 100
	Jack Knifes	4 x 15
	Feet Anchored Sit-Up	4 x 15
	Bow-to-the-Queen Lunges	4 x 15
	Stationary Bottom-Range Pulse Lunge	4 x 15
	Chest on Floor Flutter Kicks	4 x 15
Day Three	Stairs	20 minutes
Day Four	Pilates 100	1 x 100
	Jack Knifes	4 x 15
	Feet Anchored Sit-Up	4 x 15
	Bow-to-the-Queen Lunges	4 x 15
	Stationary Bottom-Range Pulse Lunge	4 x 15
	Chest on Floor Flutter Kicks	4 x 15
Day Five	Stairs	20 minutes
Day Six	Pilates 100	1 x 100
	Jack Knifes	4 x 15
	Feet Anchored Sit-Up	4 x 15
	Bow-to-the-Queen Lunges	4 x 15
	Stationary Bottom-Range Pulse Lunge	4 x 15
	Chest on Floor Flutter Kicks	4 x 15

Week Twelve

We fix things when they're broken. We worry about the sky after we've ruined the atmosphere. We enact fishing quotas after the fish are gone. We blame our leaders after we've elected them. And we worry about our health and fitness after almost 70 percent of the country is overweight or obese. We can do better—start with yourself.

DAY	EXERCISE	DURATION/ SETS & REPS
Day One	Stairs	20 minutes
Day Two	Pilates 100	1 x 100
	Jack Knifes	4 x 15
	Feet Anchored Sit-Up	4 x 15
	Bow-to-the-Queen Lunges	4 x 15
	Stationary Bottom-Range Pulse Lunge	4 x 15
	Chest on Floor Flutter Kicks	4 x 15
Day Three	Stairs	20 minutes
Day Four	Pilates 100	1 x 100
	Jack Knifes	4 x 15
	Feet Anchored Sit-Up	4 x 15
	Bow-to-the-Queen Lunges	4 x 15
	Stationary Bottom-Range Pulse Lunge	4 x 15
	Chest on Floor Flutter Kicks	4 x 15
Day Five	Stairs	20 minutes
Day Six	Pilates 100	1 x 100
	Jack Knifes	4 x 15
	Feet Anchored Sit-Up	4 x 15
	Bow-to-the-Queen Lunges	4 x 15
	Stationary Bottom-Range Pulse Lunge	4 x 15
	Chest on Floor Flutter Kicks	4 x 15

"There are admirable potentialities in every human being. Believe in your strength and your youth. Learn to repeat endlessly to yourself, 'It all depends on me.'"

—ANDRE GIDE (1869–1951)

The Final "Dirty" Thirty (Weeks Thirteen to Sixteen)

The final lap! If you were in a track race, this would be the final quarter mile. This is where the "cream separates from the milk." I also refer to the last thirty days of the program as the "rhino thirty" because this is often when you just have to put your head down and *do it*! Don't think, don't question, and don't stop! Just get up and get it done.

The final thirty days of the Butt & Gut Program is also the most intense. You're now busting your butt on the stairs for twenty minutes, three times a week, and you're also out of bed every other morning and torturing your butt and gut. It hurts and you're sore. That, my friend, is the nature of the beast—it's both the worst and the best of why you're taking this journey. And it is precisely why at this point you cannot stop the program: you've invested too much and worked too hard. Don't cash in your chips now; the best is yet to come. Rhino through!

The Final Thirty Days

- Increase your repetitions from fifteen to twenty
- Maintain your total stairs time of twenty minutes
- Rest *only* twenty seconds between sets
- Complete each workout in twenty minutes
- *Don't quit!*

Week Thirteen

Quit worrying about how much weight you'll lose and how fast. It will happen—it's not magic, it's math. Make better eating choices and exercise regularly and you'll lose weight. Weight loss isn't about a certain pill or supplement, nor does it have anything to do with a particular piece of equipment. You'll lose weight and get in shape when you decide to and not one day sooner.

DAY	EXERCISE	DURATION/ SETS & REPS
Day One	Stairs	20 minutes
Day Two	Bicycles	4 x 20
	Sumo Stance Alternate Toe Touch	4 x 20
	Seated Knee Tucks	4 x 20
	Body-Weight Squat	4 x 20
	Stationary Lunge with Straight Rear Leg	4 x 20
	Frogs	4 x 20
Day Three	Stairs	20 minutes
Day Four	Bicycles	4 x 20
	Sumo Stance Alternate Toe Touch	4 x 20
	Seated Knee Tucks	4 x 20
	Body-Weight Squat	4 x 20
	Stationary Lunge with Straight Rear Leg	4 x 20
	Frogs	4 x 20
Day Five	Stairs	20 minutes
Day Six	Bicycles	4 x 20
	Sumo Stance Alternate Toe Touch	4 x 20
	Seated Knee Tucks	4 x 20
	Body-Weight Squat	4 x 20
	Stationary Lunge with Straight Rear Leg	4 x 20
	Frogs	4 x 20

Week Fourteen

This is a long, slow voyage. Not something you want to hear? Sorry, but somebody needs to tell you the truth. Meet Mr. Somebody. I am not going to tell you that you can lose a dress size in ten days or fifty pounds in four weeks. Getting in shape and losing weight takes time and effort. It's true—nothing worth having happens quickly or easily.

DAY	EXERCISE	DURATION/ SETS & REPS
Day One	Stairs	20 minutes
Day Two	Bicycles	4 x 20
	Sumo Stance Alternate Toe Touch	4 x 20
	Seated Knee Tucks	4 x 20
	Body-Weight Squat	4 x 20
	Stationary Lunge with Straight Rear Leg	4 x 20
	Frogs	4 x 20
Day Three	Stairs	20 minutes
Day Four	Bicycles	4 x 20
	Sumo Stance Alternate Toe Touch	4 x 20
	Seated Knee Tucks	4 x 20
	Body-Weight Squat	4 x 20
	Stationary Lunge with Straight Rear Leg	4 x 20
	Frogs	4 x 20
Day Five	Stairs	20 minutes
Day Six	Bicycles	4 x 20
	Sumo Stance Alternate Toe Touch	4 x 20
	Seated Knee Tucks	4 x 20
	Body-Weight Squat	4 x 20
	Stationary Lunge with Straight Rear Leg	4 x 20
	Frogs	4 x 20

Week Fifteen

Hooray, you're doing it! You're exercising every day and making better food choices. And it's working—you feel better and you probably look better. People are noticing and because what you're doing is contagious. You're influencing your co-workers, your wife or husband, and your kids. You are a role model, displaying success and providing leadership.

DAY	EXERCISE	DURATION/ SETS & REPS
Day One	Stairs	20 minutes
Day Two	Arms at Side, Legs Bent V-Ups	4 x 20
	Reach-Through Pulse Crunch	4 x 20
	Combination Crunch and Hip Roll	4 x 20
	Lunge Wheel	4 x 20
	Narrow Stance Chair Squat	4 x 20
	Single-Leg Butt-Ups	4 x 20
Day Three	Stairs	20 minutes
Day Four	Combination Crunch and Hip Roll	4 x 20
	Reach-Through Pulse Crunch	4 x 20
	Pretzel	4 x 20
	Lunge Wheel	4 x 20
	Narrow Stance Chair Squat	4 x 20
	Single-Leg Butt-Ups	4 x 20
Day Five	Stairs	20 minutes
Day Six	Combination Crunch and Hip Roll	4 x 20
	Reach-Through Pulse Crunch	4 x 20
	Pretzel	4 x 20
	Lunge Wheel	4 x 20
	Narrow Stance Chair Squat	4 x 20
	Single-Leg Butt-Ups	4 x 20

Week Sixteen

The two most difficult parts of this program are the start and the finish, weeks one and sixteen. Why? Those first precarious steps take bravery and "balls," and week sixteen is difficult because you may be viewing it as the end and it's not. Week sixteen is just a step like all the rest, a step you'll be taking again and again. Don't lose your focus, maintain your resolve, and press on.

DAY	EXERCISE	DURATION/ SETS & REPS
Day One	Stairs	20 minutes
Day Two	Combination Crunch and Hip Roll	4 x 20
	Reach-Through Pulse Crunch	4 x 20
	Pretzel	4 x 20
	Lunge Wheel	4 x 20
	Narrow Stance Chair Squat	4 x 20
	Single-Leg Butt-Ups	4 x 20
Day Three	Stairs	20 minutes
Day Four	Combination Crunch and Hip Roll	4 x 20
	Reach-Through Pulse Crunch	4 x 20
	Pretzel	4 x 20
	Lunge Wheel	4 x 20
	Narrow Stance Chair Squat	4 x 20
	Single-Leg Butt-Ups	4 x 20
Day Five	Stairs	20 minutes
Day Six	Combination Crunch and Hip Roll	4 x 20
	Reach-Through Pulse Crunch	4 x 20
	Pretzel	4 x 20
	Lunge Wheel	4 x 20
	Narrow Stance Chair Squat	4 x 20
	Single-Leg Butt-Ups	4 x 20

*"If you greatly desire something, have the guts
to stake everything on obtaining it."*

—BRENDAN FRANCIS

Measure This?

Clients come to me all the time and *tell me* how much they'd like to weigh. It's a statement I love because I simply ask them, "Why?" Most people can't answer. The few that do usually say, "Because that's the weight I feel best at," which prompts me to ask, "How do you know?" This is where I typically stump them. The simple fact is that most of you don't know how much you should weigh, nor do most of you know what any of your various body measurements should be. So, should you be concerned?

I am not a huge fan of taking body measurements, whatever those measurements may be. I think the circumference of your hips, belly, thighs, arms, or even what you weigh are moot points. Of much more concern is that you get regular and consistent exercise. Setting a measurable physical goal is one of the principal problems with almost all of the various weight loss, health, and fitness programs available today. Let's face it, you can set all the measurable goals you want—make them as small as you want or as grandiose as you can imagine—but their attainment is eventually dependent on one single thing, you.

Instead, make regular exercise your goal. Want to focus on something? Focus on getting your ass up and moving! Think about it. What happens if you begin a consistent schedule of exercise? If suddenly you decide to incorporate some form of exercise into your daily routine, your daily calorie outlay goes up. In short, you'll be burning more calories every day than before. The almost unavoidable outcome of burning more calories daily is you'll lose weight.

Now, if you couple that daily exercise with improved food choices, then you increase the likelihood of those physical changes showing even sooner. If your overall calorie consumption goes down *and* you're breaking a sweat twenty minutes a day, six days a week, then you've increased the likelihood that your weight loss will be at an even quicker pace. You're burning more calories with exercise and you're eating less food that is better for you. Again, the cumulative effect of this is that you'll lose weight.

You'll know when it happens and you'll know how much, but don't make it your focus. Quit worrying about what you measure or what you weigh. Worry about changing your eating habits. Worry about getting regular exercise, about getting consistently off your ass! When you consistently exercise and slowly begin adjusting and changing your eating habits, the rest will take care of itself.

Chapter 4

FIFTY EXERCISES FOR YOUR BUTT

"We should be taught not to wait for inspiration to start a thing. Action always generates inspiration. Inspiration seldom generates action."

—FRANK TIBOLT

The Nuts and Bolts

The Butt & Gut Program, as outlined, incorporates twenty-four butt and twenty-four gut exercises. I have listed and depicted the exercises in this chapter and the next. However, I have also included an extra twenty-six movements for both categories. Use these movements as alternatives. Throughout the program, you may select alternative exercises from the same category level to replace an exercise in which you're struggling.

Don't choose alternatives unless it's necessary. It is necessary when you are unable to carry out the movement properly either because the exercise is simply too difficult for you to perform or because you're unable to keep the necessary form. Both are the result of your conditioning and as your fitness improves, you'll begin to master more difficult exercises.

Don't quickly decide to change exercises. More often than not, the exercise is simply hard and you're looking for an "easier" alternative. Push yourself and try not to jump ship on exercises too quickly. Changing your fitness level is hard. Don't seek shortcuts, because they don't exist. Instead, embrace difficult movements as challenges and seek to improve your performance.

*"It is amazing how much crisper the general experience
of life becomes when your body is given a chance
to develop a little strength."*

—FRANK DUFF

Exercise Tips

All the movements outlined and depicted below primarily exercise your derriere. I am providing you with fifty movements, grouped into beginning, intermediate, and advanced levels. The exercises provide varying degrees of intensity.

You'll always be working your butt with these movements, but you'll also be exercising your hamstrings, quadriceps, and calves, as well as those muscles that comprise your core (abdominals and lower back). To some degree, this is a specialized program targeting specific areas, but the exercises selected and their mechanics lend themselves to multiple muscle involvement. These are "bang for your buck" exercises.

Perform the exercises *exactly* as depicted and described. Proper form should always be your top consideration when exercising. How many repetitions you reach or how many sets you do are secondary to performing the exercises correctly. Always strive to complete the repetitions as outlined, but when fatigue and lack of conditioning don't allow you to complete the exercise with proper form, it is better to do fewer right than more wrong. Always concern yourself with quality, not quantity.

BEGINNING LEVEL BUTT (BLB) EXERCISES

The following exercises are beginning level, movements that primarily only involve one joint. However, some of the exercises involve both the hip and the knee joint. I have included all of these exercises within the beginning level category because they do not place a significant load on the exerciser. Nevertheless, you'll be using these exercises to begin improving your fitness and thus allowing you to progress to more difficult, more challenging, and thus more effective exercises.

Bent-Knee Donkey Kicks (BLB-1)

How to Do It: Space your hands and knees evenly and keep your mid-section muscles (your gut) semi-flexed. Extend and press your heel upwards and back, keeping your head and neck in line with your spine. Repeat with the other leg.

Don't Forget: Don't bring your knee to your chest, but simply lower it to the point parallel with your fixed leg. Don't explode your foot up. Stay controlled—a simple 1–2 count, up and down. Don't let your lower back sag; maintain a tight, controlled core.

Alternatives: BLB-2

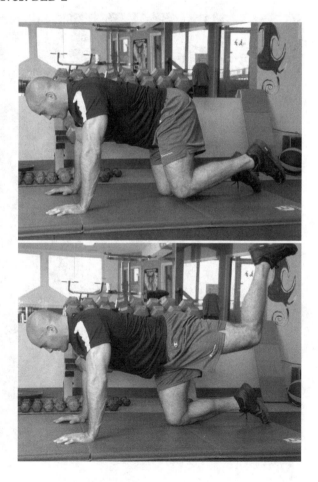

Straight-Leg Rear Raises (BLB-2)

How to Do It: Place your hands and knees evenly apart and maintain a "semi-flexed" midsection. Straighten one leg behind and point your toe. Raise your leg just above being parallel to the floor. Repeat with the other leg.

Don't Forget: Don't bring your leg too high, because doing so will cause your lower back to sag. Don't lift your head up and down; rather, maintain your head and neck in alignment with your spine. Don't lift your leg quick—keep the movement controlled.

Alternatives: BLB-1

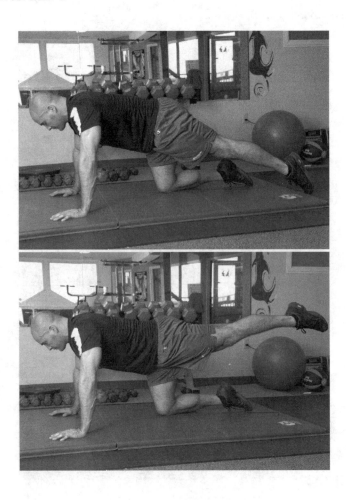

Chest on Floor Single-Leg Raises (BLB-3)

How to Do It: Lie on your chest and stomach, with your hands folded under your chin or stretched forward. Keeping your knee straight and your toes pointed away from your body, lift one leg. Return to the floor and repeat. Repeat with the other leg.

Don't Forget: Don't try to lift your leg too high—this is a short movement.

Alternatives: BLB-4, BLB-5

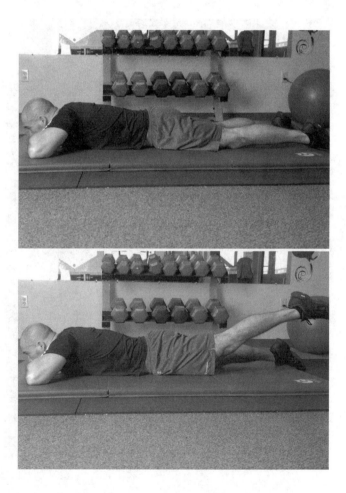

Chest on Floor Double-Leg Raises (BLB-4)

How to Do It: Perform this movement exactly as the single-leg movement (BLB-3) but with both legs simultaneously.

Don't Forget: Don't move or rock your upper body—try to remain motionless.

Alternatives: BLB-3, BLB-5

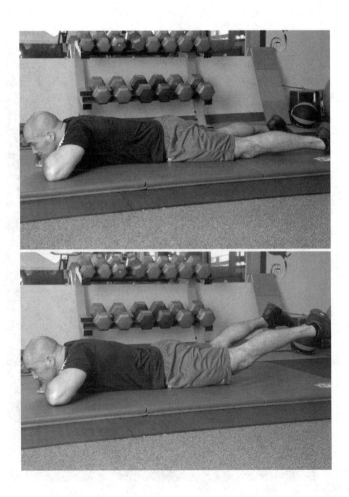

Chest on Floor Flutter Kicks (BLB-5)

How to Do It: Use the same position as the previous chest on floor leg raises (BLB-3 and BLB-4). However, instead of returning your legs to the floor between each repetition, keep the motion continuous by not completely resting your legs. While doing the exercise, imagine kicking yourself through water.

Don't Forget: Keep your toes pointed and your legs straight.

Alternatives: BLB-3, BLB-4

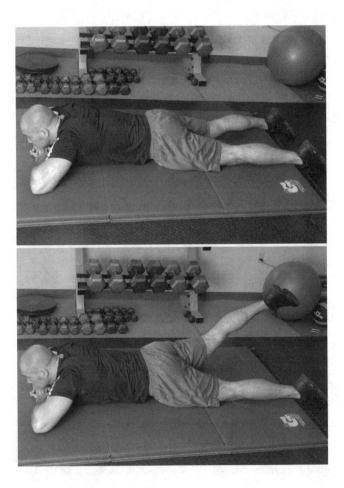

Frogs (BLB-6)

How to Do It: Lie face down and cross your arms under your chin. Keep your chest and stomach firmly on the floor. Bending your knees and turning your ankles in, press the soles of your feet together. Then, squeeze your butt and barely lift your thighs from the floor.

Don't Forget: Don't over lift or try to extend too much. This is a short, controlled movement.

Alternatives: None

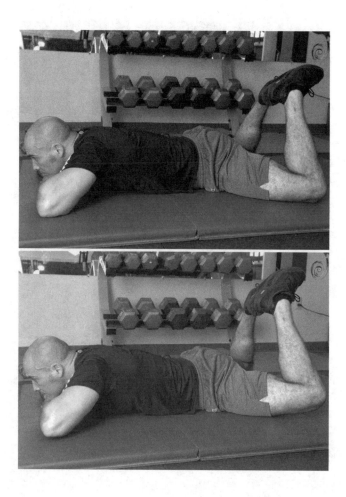

Butt-Ups (BLB-7)

How to Do It: Lie on your back with your hands at your sides. Place your feet shoulder-width apart. While keeping your head, upper back, and arms on the floor, press through your heels and extend your pelvis up. Try to lift high enough to create a straight line through your shoulders, hips, and knees.

Don't Forget: Don't drive your hips with your toes or the ball of your feet. Concentrate on pushing the force of the motion through your heels.

Alternatives: BLB-8, BLB-9, BLB-10

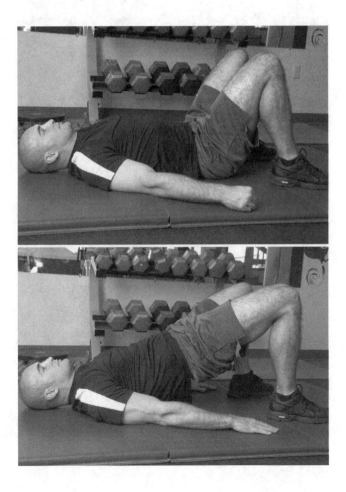

Single-Leg Butt-Ups (BLB-8)

How to Do It: From the same position as the Butt-Up (BLB-7), extend one leg. Point your toe and keep your knee straight, then drive your hips up with your one leg. Keep your other leg straight and close to the same plane as the other upper leg. Repeat with the other leg.

Don't Forget: Don't allow the raised, straight leg to rise—maintain its position with your other leg.

Alternatives: BLB-7, BLB-9, BLB-10

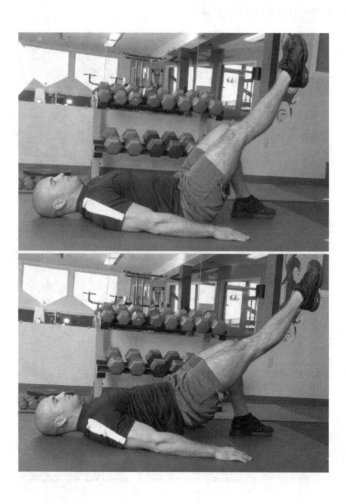

Figure Four Butt-Ups (BLB-9)

How to Do It: Cross one leg over the other in a figure four position, then drive the single leg on the floor, pressing the pelvis upwards.

Don't Forget: Don't move too quick—always maintain control throughout the motion.

Alternatives: BLB-7, BLB-8, BLB-10

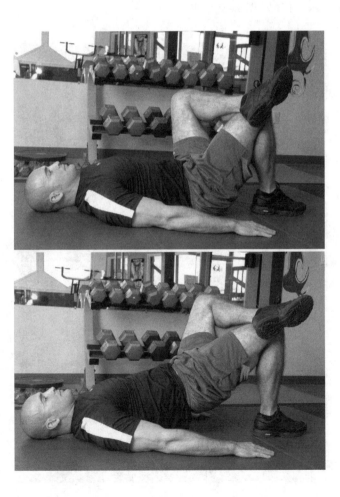

Sumo Butt-Ups with Pause (BLB-10)

How to Do It: This is the same motion as the Butt-Up (BLB-7) with the exception that you'll place your feet farther apart and exaggerate your toes pointing out. Complete a simple one-count pause at the top of each repetition. Doing so increases the intensity and aids in the continuing development of your "mind-muscle" connection.

Don't Forget: Don't allow your knees to fall to the center as you extend. Press through your heels and drive your knees out and over your toes.

Alternatives: BLB-7, BLB-8, BLB-9

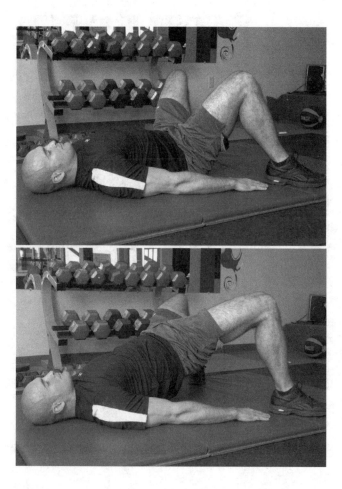

Heel in Chair Butt-Ups (BLB-11)

How to Do It: Lie on your back and place your heels on the seat of a typical table chair. Your knees should be bent at approximately 90 degrees. Then, visualize curling your heels to the back of your legs by driving your heels and lifting your hips.

Don't Forget: Maintain a "flexed" foot position.

Alternatives: BLB-12, BLB-13

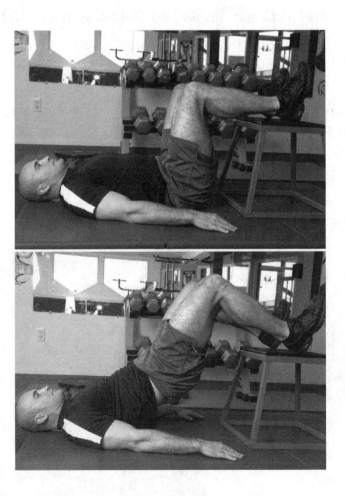

Heel in Chair Butt-Ups with Pause (BLB-12)

How to Do It: This exercise is exactly the same as the Heel in Chair Butt-Ups (BLB-11) with the exception that, once extended, you hold the position for a ten-second count, then lower and repeat.

Don't Forget: Concentrate on squeezing and tensing your glutes (butt muscles) at the point of full extension.

Alternatives: BLB-11, BLB-13

Heel in Chair Single-Leg Butt-Ups (BLB-13)

How to Do It: Perform this movement exactly as if you were performing the Single-Leg Butt-Ups (BLB-8) from the floor, except that you'll be driving your heel from a chair. Repeat with the other leg.

Don't Forget: Don't lose control of the leg you're holding straight—try to keep it in alignment with the other.

Alternatives: BLB-11, BLB-12

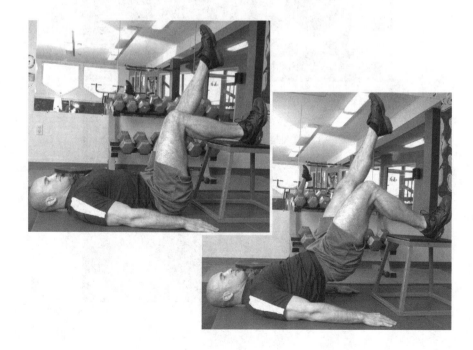

Side Leg Raise (BLB-14)

How to Do It: Lie on your side and support your head with one arm; use your other arm for balance. With a straight leg and relaxed foot, simply raise your leg as high as comfortable. Repeat with the other leg.

Don't Forget: Don't open up your hips—keep them at a 90-degree angle from the floor. If your hips are falling back, you're trying to raise your leg too high.

Alternatives: None

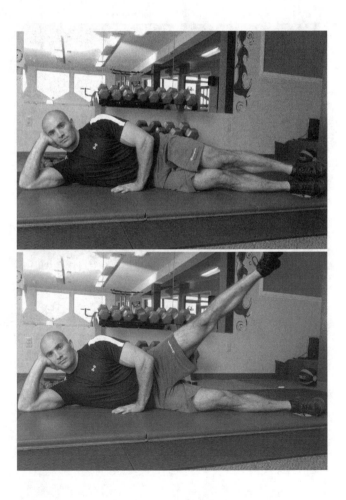

Side Leg Raise with Bent Knee (BLB-15)

How to Do It: Perform this exercise exactly as a Side Leg Raise (BLB-14) but with the exercised leg maintaining a 90-degree bend. Repeat with the other leg.

Don't Forget: Don't allow your knee to travel forward. Both knees should remain in the same alignment throughout the movement.

Alternatives: BLB-16, BLB-17

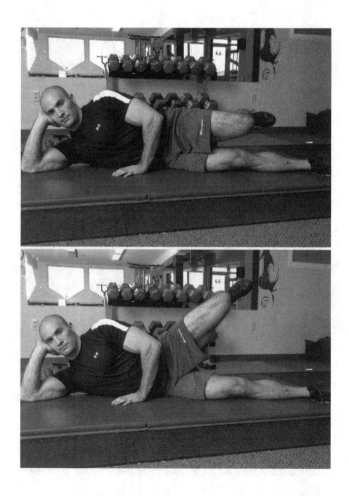

Rear Side Leg Raise (BLB-16)

How to Do It: From the Side Leg Raise (BLB-14) position, extend the leg you're exercising to the rear. Raise and lower your leg from this position. Repeat with the other leg.

Don't Forget: Don't move your leg forward as your raise it—maintain its position slightly to the rear.

Alternatives: BLB-15, BLB-17

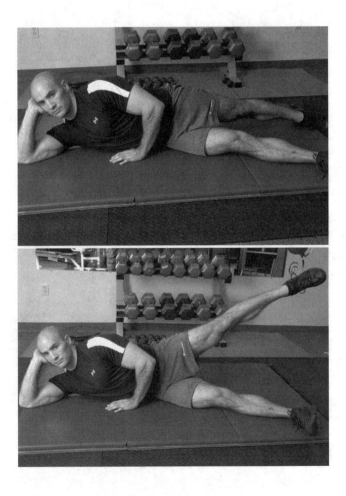

Front Side Leg Raise (BLB-17)

How to Do It: From the Side Leg Raise (BLB-14) position, extend the exercising leg to the front, then raise and lower it from this position. Repeat with the other leg.

Don't Forget: Don't point or "flex" your foot with any of the side leg raise exercises. Keep your foot relaxed.

Alternatives: BLB-15, BLB-16

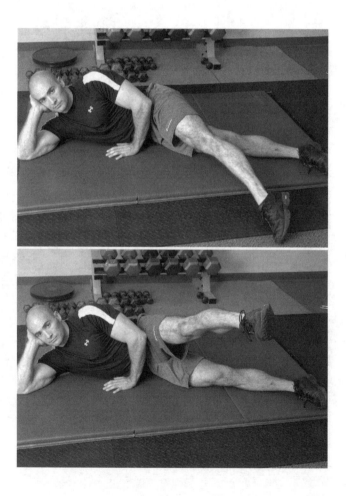

INTERMEDIATE LEVEL BUTT (ILB) EXERCISES

The intermediate level butt exercises begin to push the intensity. These are exercises that will begin putting your joints through a longer range of motion and that will substantially involve at least two joints. Remember, typically the more range we put a joint through, the higher the degree of muscle involvement. And again, that's good—the more muscles involved means a greater demand on your cardiovascular system and more calories burned. That's what you're after.

Chair Squat (ILB-1)

How to Do It: Position yourself over a typical table chair. Place the chair in a diagonal position. Stand with your feet shoulder-width (or slightly wider) apart, with your toes pointing out. Raise your arms forward, keeping them parallel with the floor. Keep your eyes facing forward and slowly lower yourself until you lightly touch the chair, then return to the standing position.

Don't Forget: Don't roll your back—concentrate on keeping your head and chest up and maintain your lower back arch. Don't press from your toes; sit back and learn to feel your body weight from your heels.

Alternatives: ILB-2, ILB-3

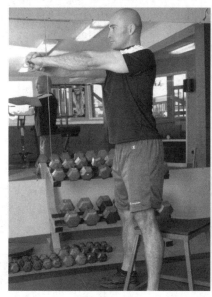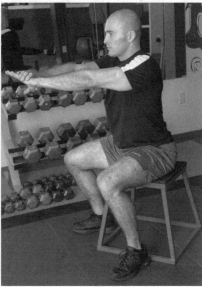

Chair Squat with Pause (ILB-2)

How to Do It: Perform this exercise exactly as the Chair Squat (ILB-1) with one difference: instead of lightly touching your rear and returning to the standing position, actually *sit* on the chair. Take all your weight off your feet, then return to the standing position.

Don't Forget: Don't drop your arms upon sitting—maintain your position. Keep your lower back arched and your chest up.

Alternatives: ILB-1, ILB-3

Feet Forward Squats (ILB-3)

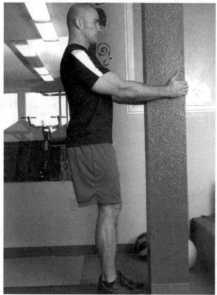

How to Do It: Grasp the knob of a closed door with both hands. Place your feet approximately four to eight inches from the door, no wider than shoulder-width apart and toes pointing straight ahead. Holding the door knob with arms straight, allow your body to lean back—your arms should feel your body weight. Then, squat down to below where your thighs are parallel to the floor and return to standing position.

Don't Forget: Don't bend your arms and don't use them to pull yourself back to a standing position. Don't lean forward—try to keep your shoulders and hips in alignment.

Alternatives: ILB-1, ILB-2

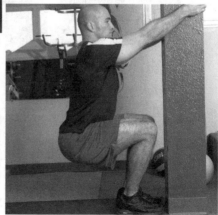

Assisted Stationary Lunge (ILB-4)

How to Do It: Place one leg forward and the other to the rear. Your rear leg should be positioned and supported by the ball of the foot. Slowly lower until your back knee lightly touches the floor. Using your front leg, drive yourself back up to the erect position. Maintain one hand on a table, chair, or ledge to assist yourself with the movement. Repeat with the other leg in the forward position.

Don't Forget: Don't allow your torso to lean forward—maintain a chest up, shoulders back position and keep your torso directly over your hips throughout the entire exercise. Don't keep your rear leg straight; allow your knee to naturally bend and fall in line with both your hip and shoulder joints at the bottom of the movement.

Alternatives: ILB-5

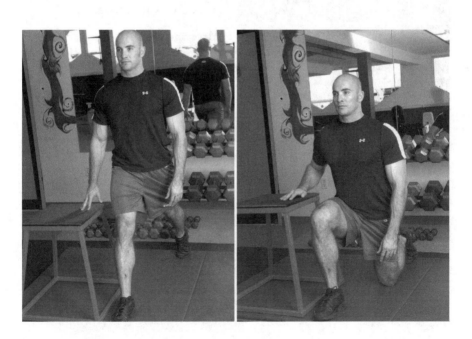

Assisted Stationary Lunge with Range Limit (ILB-5)

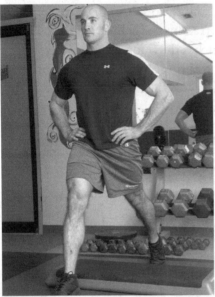

How to Do It: Perform this movement exactly as the Stationary Lunge (ILB-4), but limit the downward range of motion. Instead of taking your knee completely to the floor, limit the range to approximately 50 to 75 percent. Maintain one hand on a table, chair, or ledge to assist yourself with the movement.

Don't Forget: Don't drop into position too fast—control the exercise. Your tempo should be the same for both the upward and downward movements.

Alternatives: ILB-4

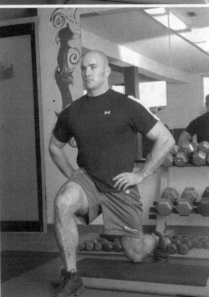

Narrow Stance Chair Squat (ILB-6)

How to Do It: Stand directly in front of a table chair. Place your feet four to six inches apart, with your toes facing directly ahead. Keep your head up and your eyes looking forward. Slowly squat down and back until your rear touches the chair, then return to standing position.

Don't Forget: Don't leave your arms at the side—raise them to the front and keep them parallel to the floor throughout the exercise.

Alternatives: ILB-7, ILB-8, ILB-9

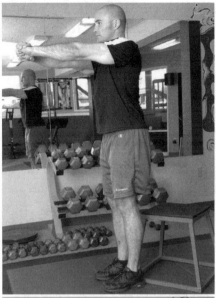

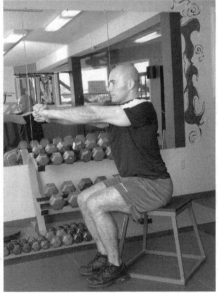

Sumo Stance Chair Squat (ILB-7)

How to Do It: Position a table chair in a diamond formation. Standing slightly over one corner of the seat, place your feet wider than shoulder-width apart with an exaggerated "toes out" stance. Slowly lower to the chair, touch, and return to a standing position.

Don't Forget: Don't allow your body weight to roll to your toes or the balls of your feet. Keep your body weight over your heels and press through them as your return to the standing position.

Alternatives: ILB-6, ILB-8, ILB-9

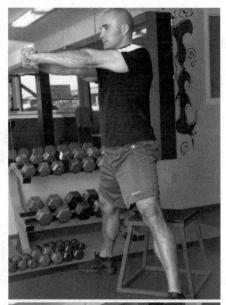

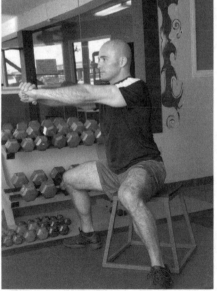

Heels Elevated Chair Squat (ILB-8)

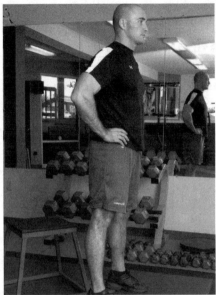

How to Do It: Position a chair in the diamond formation. Stand slightly over one corner with your feet slightly wider than shoulder-width apart. Your toes should be turned slightly and naturally out. Place a book or other flat object, approximately one inch thick, under your heels. Squat down and slightly back until you touch the chair, then return to a standing the position.

Don't Forget: Don't slouch—maintain a position with your chest up and lower back arched.

Alternatives: ILB-6, ILB-7, ILB-9

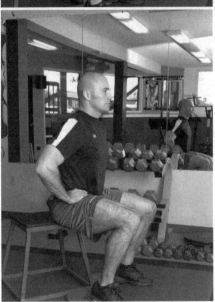

Toes Elevated Chair Squat (ILB-9)

How to Do It: This exercise is performed exactly like the Heels Elevated Chair Squat (ILB-8), except instead of elevating your heels, you'll elevate the balls of your feet. Position a book or other flat object, approximately a half inch thick (a typical magazine is usually perfect), securely under the balls of your feet. Lower yourself until you lightly touch the chair, then return to a standing position.

Don't Forget: Don't drop to the chair. Lower yourself slowly and under control at all times. Elevating your feet from the front forces your body weight onto your heels.

Alternatives: ILB-6, ILB-7, ILB-8

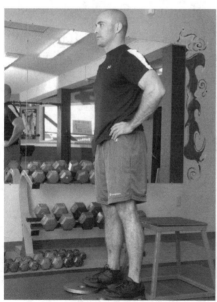 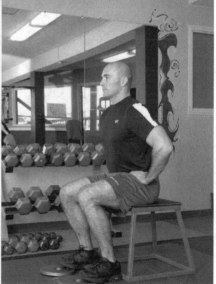

ADVANCED LEVEL BUTT (ALB) EXERCISES

The advanced level butt exercises are tough! That's the nature of the beast. These are exercises that involve long, full ranges of motion with multiple joints. These are also complex movements that require you to exercise your balance, coordination, and athleticism, which also means that your core muscles will be active and involved providing torso stabilization. We're targeting certain areas of the body, but we're doing it with exercises that provide solid, balanced body conditioning.

Body-Weight Squat (ALB-1)

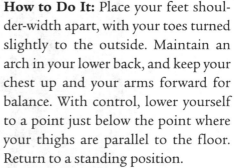

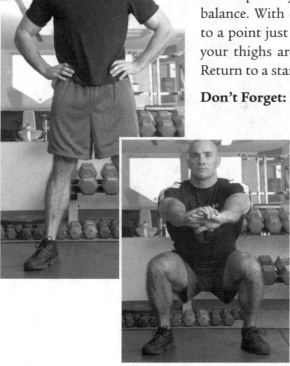

How to Do It: Place your feet shoulder-width apart, with your toes turned slightly to the outside. Maintain an arch in your lower back, and keep your chest up and your arms forward for balance. With control, lower yourself to a point just below the point where your thighs are parallel to the floor. Return to a standing position.

Don't Forget: Don't press from the balls of your feet and don't rock forward—keep your body weight on your heels.

Alternatives: None

Jump Squat (ALB-2)

How to Do It: Perform this exercise exactly as the Body-Weight Squat (ALB-1), with one substantial difference—instead of pressing from your heels and returning to the starting position, initiate an explosive jump from the bottom position, literally jumping to your feet.

Don't Forget: Don't lose control. Explosive movements are not excuses for sloppy form.

Alternatives: ALB-3, ALB-4, ALB-5, ALB-6

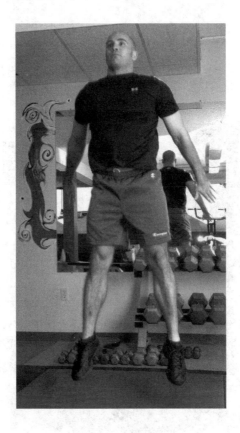

Sumo Jump Squat (ALB-3)

How to Do It: Standing upright, take a wider than normal squat stance. Place your feet in an exaggerated toes out position. With your chest up and arms forward for balance, lower yourself to the point where your thighs are parallel to the floor. Forcefully press your feet into the floor and jump to the original starting position.

Don't Forget: Don't bring your feet together after jumping. Catch yourself in the same foot and stance position. Squat, jump, and return to the same stance.

Alternatives: ALB-2, ALB-4, ALB-5, ALB-6

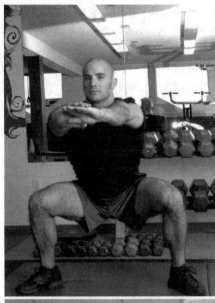

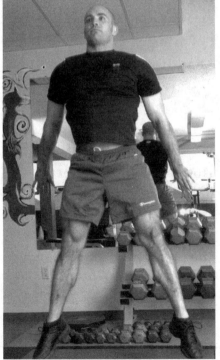

Sumo Jump Squat to Soldier Stand (ALB-4)

How to Do It: This exercise is performed almost exactly as the Sumo Jump Squat (ALB-3). In this variation, the position of your feet upon completing the jump is different. Instead of catching yourself in the sumo position, complete the exercise with your feet together. Then, simply step back to sumo position and repeat the exercise.

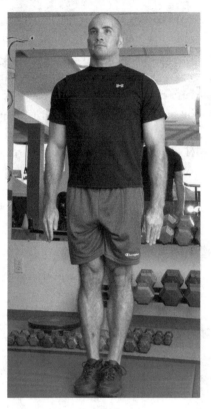

Don't Forget: Don't be in hurry with this exercise. Maintain control, position, and form throughout. Don't underestimate the intensity of your jump—returning to a feet-together position requires slightly more force in order to achieve the height necessary.

Alternatives: ALB-2, ALB-3, ALB-5, ALB-6

Jump to Squat (ALB-5)

How to Do It: With feet shoulder-width apart, perform a moderate-intensity jump and catch yourself in the bottom position of the squat. With chest up and lower back arched, press through your heels and return to the upright position.

Don't Forget: Don't simply drop to the bottom of the squat after your jump—the motion should be a controlled fall. Maintain a tight core and semi-flexed legs to act as shock absorbers.

Alternatives: ALB-2, ALB-3, ALB-4, ALB-6

Hands-Behind-Head Squat (ALB-6)

How to Do It: Perform this exercise exactly as you would perform the Body-Weight Squat (ALB-1), with one difference: place your hands (with fingers locked together) behind your head.

Don't Forget: Don't allow your elbows to face forward—keep your chest up and your elbows pointed outward over your shoulders. Don't pull on your head; keep your arms behind your head without applying pressure. Also, don't lean forward. Placing your hands behind your head changes your center of gravity and potentially makes the motion more difficult.

Alternatives: ALB-2, ALB-3, ALB-4, ALB-5

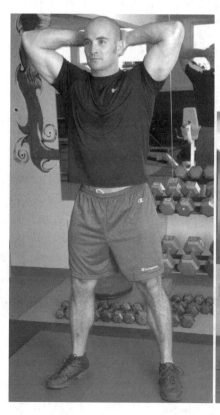
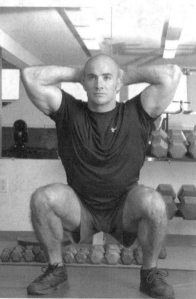

Toe Squat (ALB-7)

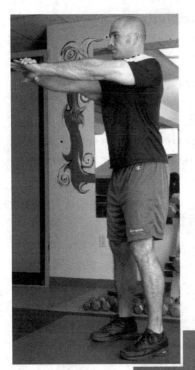

How to Do It: Stand with feet shoulder-width apart and extend your arms forward for balance. Drive your knees forward and drop your hips directly to your heels. Press from the balls of your feet back to slowly return to a feet flat, standing position.

Don't Forget: Don't press from your heels. The bottom position of this squat variation places your body weight precariously on the balls of your feet. It is very much an exercise in strength and balance.

Alternatives: None

Single-Leg Squat (ALB-8)

How to Do It: Stand on one leg with chest up and arms at your sides. Slowly lower your chest to your knee while reaching for the floor. Touch the floor and press yourself back to the upright position. Repeat with the other leg.

Don't Forget: Don't lean too far forward. At the bottom of the position, your chin should be slightly forward of your knee. Don't press from the front of your foot—you should feel your body weight on your heels. Use your other leg for balance by extending it to the rear.

Alternatives: None

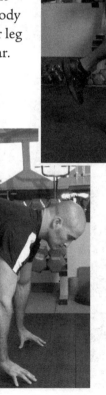

Stationary Lunge (ALB-9)

How to Do It: Standing erect, place one foot slightly forward and flat on the floor; place your other leg to the rear, positioned on the ball of the foot. Maintain an erect torso over your hips throughout the motion. Slowly lower yourself until the knee of the rear leg lightly touches the floor, then press, returning to the starting position. At the bottom position of the movement, both of your knees should demonstrate a minimum 90-degree bend. Repeat with the other leg forward.

Don't Forget: Don't extend your rear leg too far. At the bottom position, your rear leg's knee should be in line with both your hip joint and your shoulders.

Alternatives: ALB-10, ALB-11

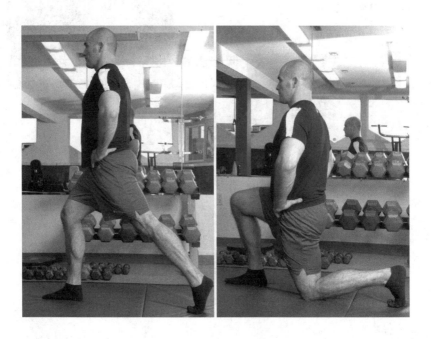

Stationary Bottom-Range Pulse Lunge (ALB-10)

How to Do It: Position yourself exactly as you would for a Stationary Lunge (ALB-9). However, instead of pressing to a full extended position, the motion is limited to the bottom range only. Once your rear knee lightly touches the floor, press yourself up approximately one-third of the total range, then return to the bottom position and repeat. Repeat with the other leg forward.

Don't Forget: Don't be too quick with this motion; keep it slow and controlled at all times.

Alternatives: ALB-9, ALB-11

Stationary Lunge with Straight Rear Leg (ALB-11)

How to Do It: This lunge variation is different because your rear leg is extended to a full-length position, which is maintained throughout the exercise. Slowly lower yourself until your front knee is bent at approximately 90 degrees, then return to a full upright position.

Don't Forget: Don't lean forward—keep your torso upright and your weight centered over your hips. As with squats, always press from your heels.

Alternatives: ALB-9, ALB-10

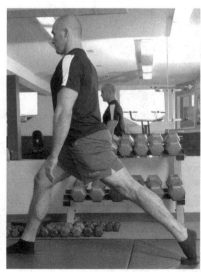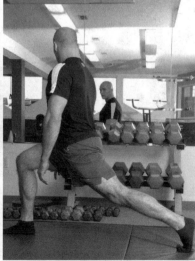

Step Back Lunge (ALB-12)

How to Do It: Stand fully upright with arms to your sides, chest up, and shoulders back. Your feet should be placed shoulder-width apart. In a smooth, controlled motion, step back and securely place your rear leg on the ball of your foot, then lower until your knee lightly touches the floor. With a controlled motion, press your front leg driving your torso upright and returning your rear leg to the initial starting position. Repeat with the other leg stepping back.

Don't Forget: Don't rush this movement, as it is complex with multiple parts. Take your time and learn to understand the mechanics of the motion.

Alternatives: ALB-13, ALB-14, ALB-15, ALB-16, ALB-17

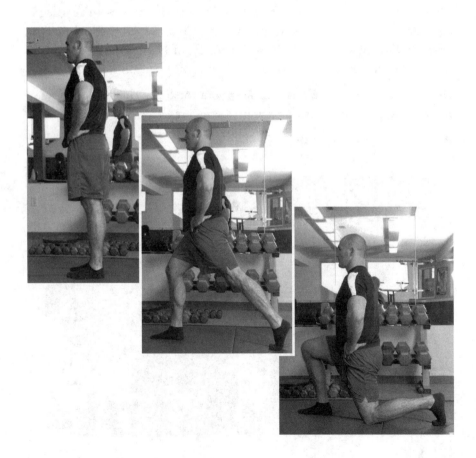

Step Back Lunge with Pull Through (ALB-13)

How to Do It: Start this movement exactly as the Step Back Lunge (ALB-12). Slowly lower yourself, lightly touching the knee, and press upright. Then, lift the rear leg, and pull through and raise your thigh until it is parallel to the floor. Pause, then return the raised leg to the rear and repeat. Repeat with the other leg.

Don't Forget: Don't get frustrated with this movement. This is an exercise that relies heavily on balance, which, like all motor skills, is dependent on usage. Use it or lose it.

Alternatives: ALB-12, ALB-14, ALB-15, ALB-16, ALB-17

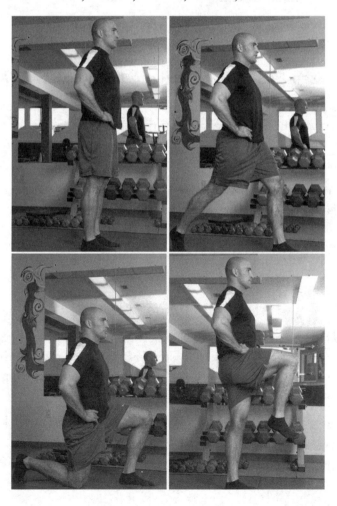

Step Forward Lunge (ALB-14)

How to Do It: The opposite of the Step Back Lunge (ALB-12), with this variation you step forward instead. Taking a reasonable stride forward, securely place your foot and drop the knee of your rear leg lightly to the floor. Press explosively from the heel, maintaining an upright torso, and return to a standing upright position. Repeat stepping forward with the other leg.

Don't Forget: Don't allow your body weight to lean forward as you step. Keep your body positioned securely over your hips, with your chest up and your shoulders back.

Alternatives: ALB-12, ALB-13, ALB-15, ALB-16, ALB-17

Step Back, Step Forward Lunge (ALB-15)

How to Do It: This exercise is a merger of both the Step Back Lunge (ALB-12) and the Step Forward Lunge (ALB-14). Perform both movements as described above, alternating the motion from front to back with the same leg. Repeat with the other leg.

Don't Forget: Don't lose awareness of where your torso and your body weight are during the movement. Keep your center of gravity securely over your hips.

Alternatives: ALB-12, ALB-13, ALB-14, ALB-16, ALB-17

Walking Lunge (ALB-16)

How to Do It: The Walking Lunge is performed similarly to the Step Forward Lunge (ALB-14). However, instead of pressing back into the standing position, you press up into the standing position, then repeat with the other leg.

Don't Forget: Don't forget to always press through your heel, keeping your chest up and torso over your hips.

Alternatives: ALB-12, ALB-13, ALB-14, ALB-15, ALB-17

Hands-Behind-Head Lunge (ALB-17)

How to Do It: This exercise is performed exactly as the Stationary Lunge (ALB-9), with the exception that your hands are placed behind your head, with the fingers locked. Repeat with the other leg forward.

Don't Forget: Don't let your elbows face forward—press them back and over your shoulders, keeping your chest up.

Alternatives: ALB-12, ALB-13, ALB-14, ALB-15, ALB-16

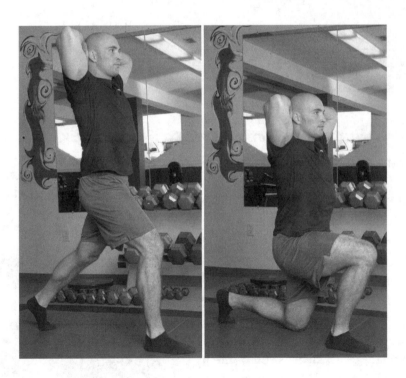

Stationary Jump Lunge (ALB-18)

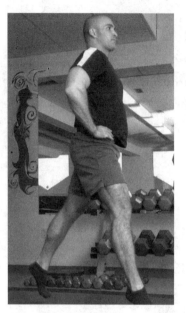

How to Do It: Assuming the Stationary Lunge (ALB-9) position, slowly lower until the knee of your rear leg lightly touches the floor. Explosively press upwards, driving both your front leg and rear leg off the floor a few inches. Press and catch yourself in the lunge stance. Repeat with the other leg.

Don't Forget: Don't allow your foot position to change upon completing the jump. Lower yourself and jump with the same foot stance.

Alternatives: ALB-19, ALB-20

Stationary Jump Lunge to Stand (ALB-19)

How to Do It: Perform this movement exactly as the Stationary Jump Lunge (ALB-18). However, instead of performing a shallow jump, maintaining your foot placement, explode hard off the floor and launch yourself up into an upright standing position. Step back into the lunge position and repeat. Repeat with the other leg.

Don't Forget: Don't leave your arms at your sides. Use them as you would if jumping onto a platform, driving your arms forcefully up as you explode from the floor.

Alternatives: ALB-18, ALB-20

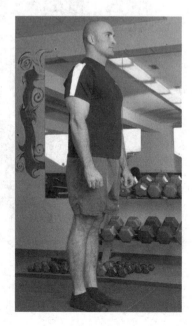

Jump Scissor Lunge (ALB-20)

How to Do It: From the bottom of the Stationary Lunge (ALB-9) position, explode up aggressively. In mid air, scissor your legs switching their position. Upon landing in the lunge position, repeat the motion.

Don't Forget: Don't be intimidated by this complex motion. This may be the most difficult of all the butt exercises, but don't let that discourage you. Aspire to master this exercise.

Alternatives: ALB-18, ALB-19

Ski Lunge (ALB-21)

How to Do It: Stand with feet together, arms at your sides, and upright. Keeping your toes pointed forward, take a large step to the side. Keeping your back flat and twisting your torso, bring your opposing elbow to your bent knee. Forcefully drive from the outside, returning yourself to the starting position.

Don't Forget: Don't simply bend at the waist and touch your elbow to your knee. Keep your back arched and press your hips to the rear.

Alternatives: ALB-22

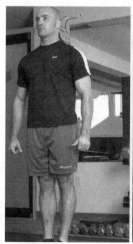
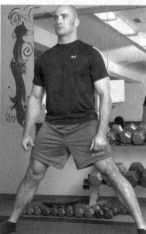
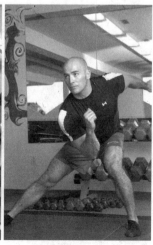

Ski Lunge with Bunny Hop (ALB-22)

How to Do It: From the Ski Lunge (ALB-21) position, and upon driving yourself back to the upright starting position, perform a short bunny hop, then repeat the lunge to the other side.

Don't Forget: Don't underestimate the significance of the bunny hop. This short, seemingly inconsequential movement will raise your heart rate considerably.

Alternatives: ALB-21

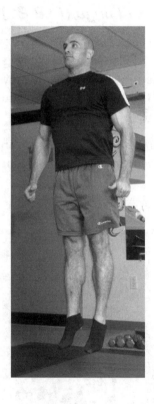

Bow-to-the-Queen Lunge (ALB-23)

How to Do It: Stand upright with your feet shoulder-width apart, your chest up, and your shoulders back. Take a lunge step forward. Lower your chest to your knee, placing your chin just forward of your bent knee. Lightly touch your hands and your back knee to the floor, press back aggressively, and repeat. Repeat with the other leg.

Don't Forget: Don't worry about maintaining an arched back—allow your back to comfortably roll over while placing your chest on your thigh. Both knees should be bent at approximately 90 degrees at the bottom position.

Alternatives: None

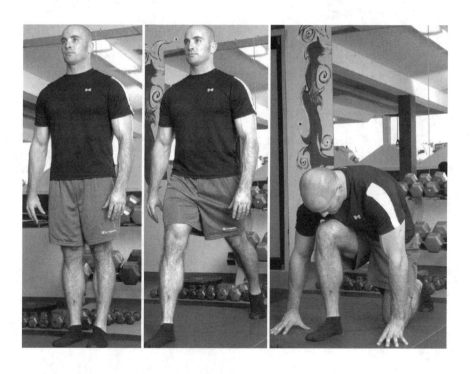

Lunge Wheel (ALB-24)

How to Do It: Start by stepping forward, performing a Bow-to-the-Queen Lunge (ALB-23). Press back aggressively, then step to your right, performing a Ski Lunge (ALB-21). Drive aggressively back to the center, then perform a Step Back Lunge (ALB-12). Once again, return to the starting position, then step to the other side for one last ski lunge.

Don't Forget: Don't hurry—take your time with these movements; it's not a race.

Alternatives: None

Chapter 5

FIFTY EXERCISES FOR YOUR GUT

*"Determine never to be idle . . . It is wonderful how much
may be done if we are always doing."*
—THOMAS JEFFERSON (1743–1826)

I have selected the gut exercises in the Butt & Gut Program with similar criteria as the butt exercises. We start with simple movements that to some degree provide limited muscle isolation. Then, as the program progresses, you'll use more advanced movements that will need added accessory muscle action. The more muscles we involve, the more intense the exercise. More muscle movement needs more energy and that places a greater demand on your body's physiology—your heart pumps faster and you breathe harder. However, it is the design of your body's midsection that makes it almost impossible to "single out" certain muscles. Maybe more so than anywhere else in the body, the muscles that comprise your midsection and your core work in an interconnected fashion. We can vary the degree of muscle involvement with exercise selection, but we cannot isolate.

BEGINNING LEVEL GUT (BLG) EXERCISES

The movements outlined in this section are foundational to all the other gut exercises you'll learn and complete. They are simple, effective movements that will strengthen your core, teach you muscle control, and prepare you for more advanced and more difficult exercises.

Basic Crunch (BLG-1)

How to Do It: Lie on your back with your hands behind your head and fingers clasped together, your knees bent, and your feet flat on the floor. With your chin up and elbows held out in a stationary position, roll your shoulders up. As your shoulders rise, press your sternum down and your lower back into the floor.

Don't Forget: Don't pull on your head. Instead, focus on contracting your midsection muscles.

Alternatives: BLG-2, BLG-3, BLG-4, BLG-7

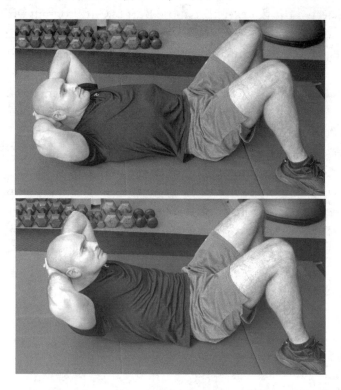

Lower Back Supported Crunch (BLG-2)

How to Do It: Lying on your back, place your hands (palms down) under the small of your back. Slowly roll you head and shoulder up and off the floor. Your elbows should be free from the floor at the highest point of the motion.

Don't Forget: Don't drop your chin—keep your chin up and stationary throughout the movement.

Alternatives: BLG-1, BLG-3, BLG-4, BLG-7

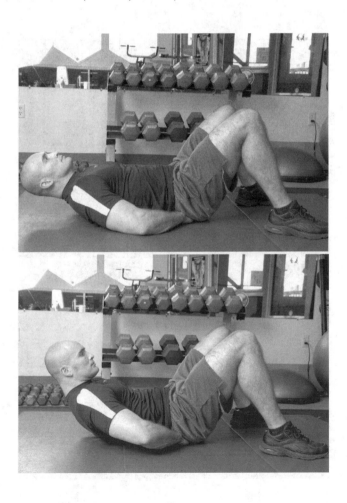

Shin Touch Crunch (BLG-3)

How to Do It: Start from the Basic Crunch (BLG-1) position. With your arms at your sides and palms facing toward your body, slowly roll your torso and reach for the outsides of your shins. Lower and repeat the motion.

Don't Forget: Don't try to make the crunch motion longer than it is. The Basic Crunch and its variations are short, tight motions.

Alternatives: BLG-1, BLG-2, BLG-4, BLG-7

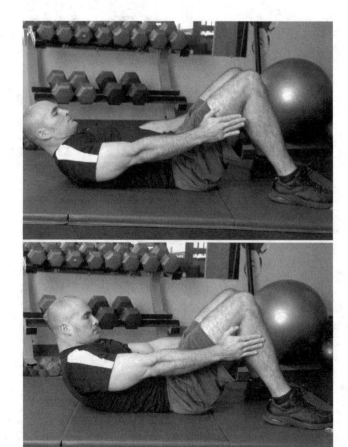

Frog Crunch (BLG-4)

How to Do It: Lying on your back, draw your heels up toward your torso until the soles of your feet are flat against one another. With hands clasped behind your head, perform the Basic Crunch (BLG-1) motion.

Don't Forget: Don't overarch your lower back—try to minimize its movement throughout the exercise.

Alternatives: BLG-1, BLG-2, BLG-3, BLG-7

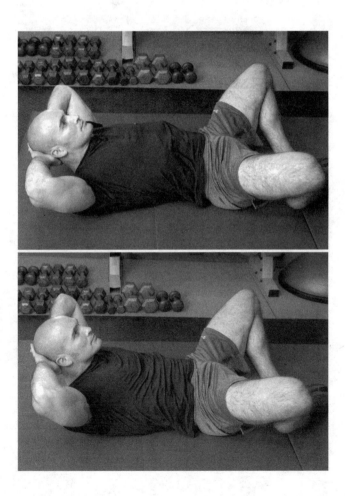

Arms Extended Crunch (BLG-5)

How to Do It: From the position of the Basic Crunch (BLG-1), place your arms extended, clasped back, and over your midsection. Reach through your legs as you crunch.

Don't Forget: Don't jerk your arms forward with this motion. Keep your arms stationary and try not to create momentum.

Alternatives: BLG-1, BLG-2, BLG-3, BLG-4

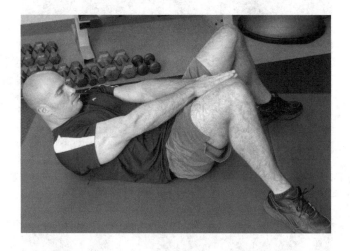

Side Crunch (BLG-6)

How to Do It: Lie on your side; clasp the free arm behind your head and point your elbow up. Slowly roll your torso toward your hips, then lower and repeat. Repeat lying on your other side.

Don't Forget: Don't believe this exercise is the secret to ridding yourself of fat that has accumulated on your sides ("love handles"). This exercise (like any) cannot reduce or remove fat from specific areas.

Alternatives: None

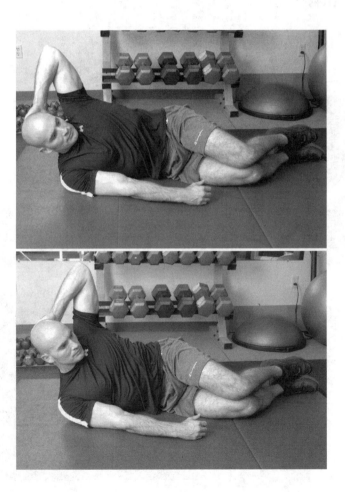

Hip Crunch (BLG-7)

How to Do It: Lie on your back with your arms to your sides, resting your arms and head on the floor. Cross your feet at the ankle and raise them off the ground. Maintain your head and shoulders securely on the ground and slowly roll your hips up and toward your head.

Don't Forget: Don't allow your legs to roll ahead of your hips. Doing so takes advantage of leverage and decreases the effectiveness of the exercise.

Alternatives: None

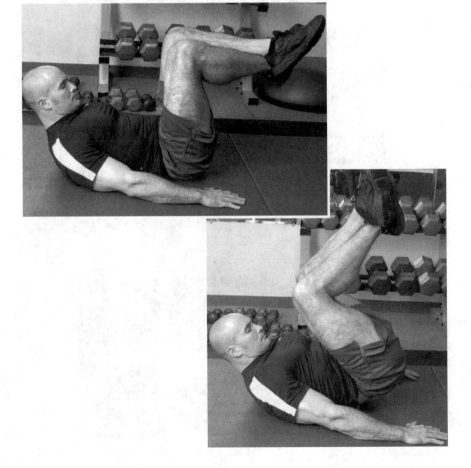

Standing Stomach Vacuum (BLG-8)

How to Do It: Stand fully erect with your chest up and shoulders back. Place your hands either at your sides or on your hips. Pull your belly button inward toward your spine as far as you can. Relax and repeat.

Don't Forget: Don't underestimate the significance of this movement—it works a set of muscles located inside your abdominal cavity against your spine. Once strengthened, these muscles provide necessary support and stability to your lower back.

Alternatives: BLG-9, BLG-10

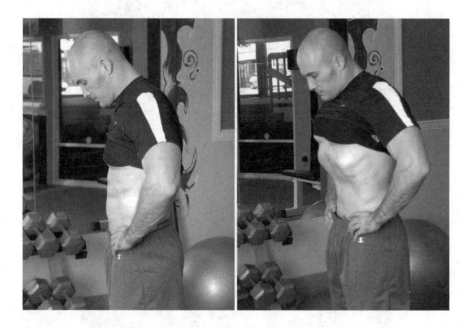

Lying Stomach Vacuum (BLG-9)

How to Do It: Lie on your back in the Basic Crunch (BLG-1) position and pull your abdominals inward. This variation of the stomach vacuum takes advantage of gravity, allowing you more ease to pull your exterior abdominals inward toward your spine.

Don't Forget: Don't raise your head and shoulders—keep them securely on the floor throughout the exercise.

Alternatives: BLG-8, BLG-10

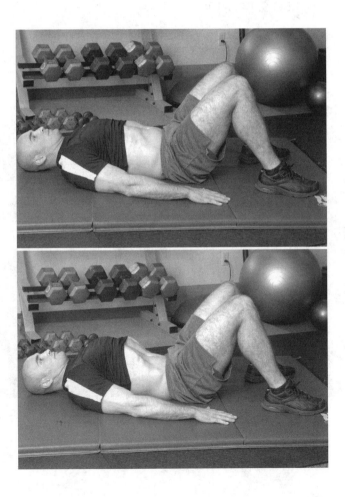

All Fours Stomach Vacuum (BLG-10)

How to Do It: Assume an "all fours" position, spacing your hands and knees evenly. Then, slowly draw your belly button inward toward your spine. Relax and repeat.

Don't Forget: Maintain a neutral back position throughout the motion—do not allow your lower back to sag as your abdominals relax.

Alternatives: BLG-8, BLG-9

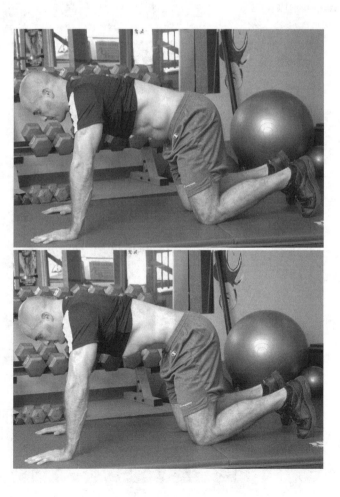

Single-Leg Raise (BLG-11)

How to Do It: Lie on your back with your arms to the sides and on the floor. Place your legs straight, with one leg raised approximately twelve inches and the other stationary on the ground. Lift the raised leg until perpendicular with the floor. Lower and repeat. Repeat with the other leg.

Don't Forget: Don't leave your head and shoulders on the floor. Instead roll your head and shoulders off the floor and maintain them in this position throughout the exercise.

Alternatives: BLG-12

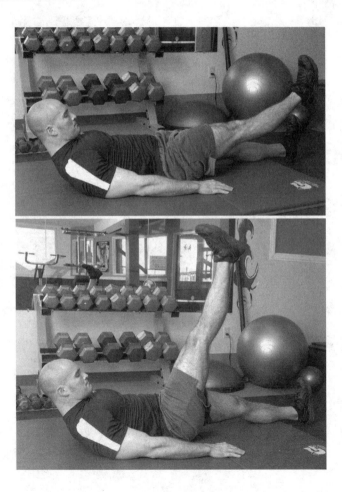

Leg Raise (BLG-12)

How to Do It: Lie flat on your back, with arms at your sides and on the floor. Legs are held together, extended, and approximately twelve inches off the floor. With your head and shoulders slightly rolled up from the floor, raise both legs together until perpendicular with the floor.

Don't Forget: Don't forget to keep your head and shoulders slightly off the floor. Doing so activates your upper abdominals and keeps them involved in the motion.

Alternatives: BLG-11

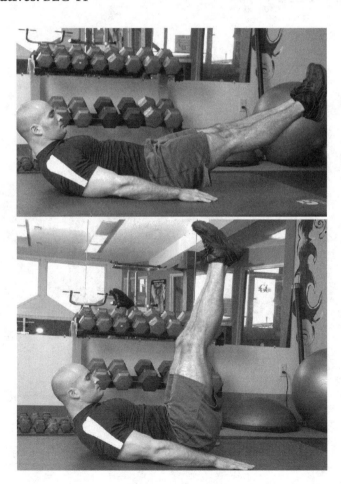

Hip Roll (BLG-13)

How to Do It: Lie on your back, legs extended and together, approximately twelve inches off the ground. Slowly pull your knees inward toward your torso and, with control, roll your hips up and slightly forward. Return and repeat.

Don't Forget: Don't pull your knees inward too quickly. Doing so would take advantage of momentum and make the movement less effective.

Alternatives: BLG-14

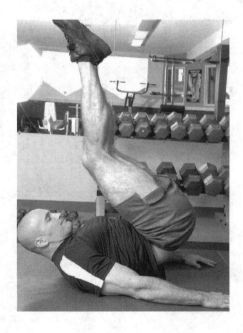

Hip Lift (BLG-14)

How to Do It: Lie on your back and place your legs together and extended upwards, perpendicular to the floor. Lift your feet upwards, then lower and repeat.

Don't Forget: Don't lift your feet back and toward your head. Press them upwards by lifting your hips and squeezing your abdominals.

Alternatives: BLG-12

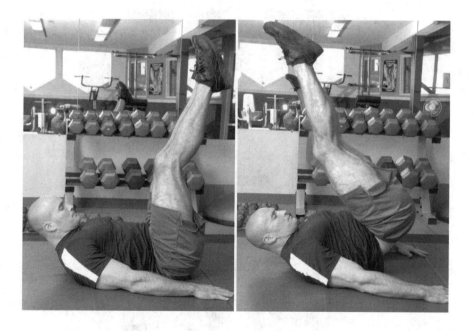

Seated Knee Tucks (BLG-15)

How to Do It: Sitting on your hips, lean your torso back at approximately 45 degrees and support yourself with your arms to your sides. Extend your legs outward and slightly off the floor. Slowly pull your legs inward toward your torso, simultaneously moving your upper torso forward. Maintain your balance and center of gravity over your hips.

Don't Forget: Don't relax your abdominal muscles—focus on keeping them tight throughout the motion.

Alternatives: BLG-11

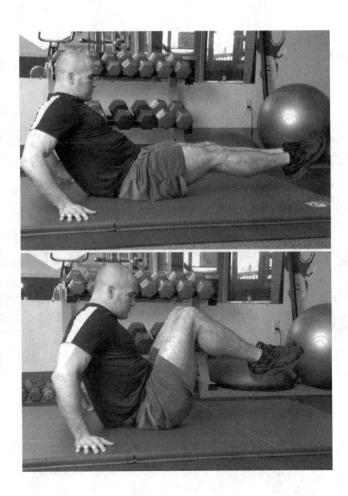

INTERMEDIATE LEVEL GUT (ILG) EXERCISES

With the gut exercises below, we begin to "raise the bar"—these exercises will challenge your physical effort as well as your execution. Simply put, these are more difficult exercises. As with every exercise in the program, remember to work hard at performing the movements with proper form. Doing an exercise incorrectly will lead to a whole host of complications, including potential injury and lack of results, both of which may cause you to become disenchanted and unmotivated. Doing the exercises in the wrong way is an avoidable step toward quitting.

Leg Raises with Hip Lift (ILG-1)

How to Do It: Lie on your back with your arms to your sides and on the floor. Your head and shoulders should be stationary and on the ground. Begin the movement with your legs straight and raised. While maintaining straight legs, raise them until they are perpendicular to the floor. Once perpendicular, lift your toes to the ceiling by lifting and rolling your hips.

Don't Forget: Do not use the momentum generated by the leg lift to carry you through the hip raise. After reaching a perpendicular position, pause for a moment before lifting and rolling your hips.

Alternatives: ILG-2

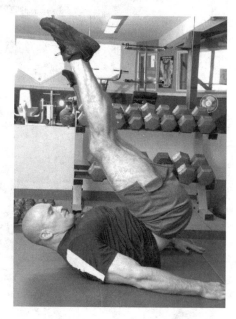

Seated Knee Tucks with Twist (ILG-2)

How to Do It: Sitting on your hips, lean your torso back at approximately 45 degrees and support yourself with your arms to your sides. Extend your legs outward and slightly off the floor. Slowly pull your legs inward while twisting your knees to the outside of your torso.

Don't Forget: Don't over twist—it is meant to be a subtle movement. Don't twist merely at the top of the motion. The twist should be executed at almost the conception of the movement.

Alternatives: ILG-1

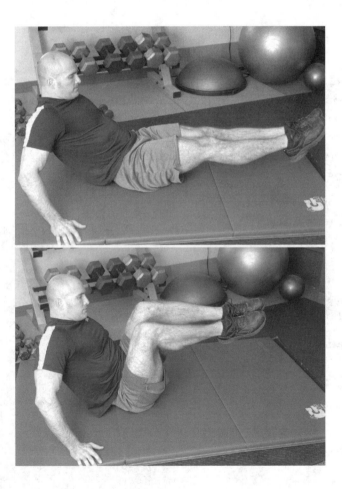

Feet Up, Ankles Crossed Crunch (ILG-3)

How to Do It: Lie on your back in the Basic Crunch (BLG-1) position. Bend your knees, then cross your ankles and raise them off the floor. With hands clasped behind your head and elbows out, slowly roll your head and shoulders off the floor. Throughout the motion, maintain your legs in the lifted and crossed position.

Don't Forget: Don't allow your elbows to travel inward; hold them out and over your shoulders, paying careful attention to not pull on the back of your head.

Alternatives: ILG-4, ILG-5, ILG-6, ILG-7, ILG-8, ILG-9

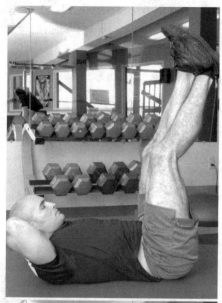

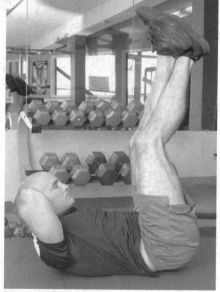

Legs Straight and Crossed Crunch (ILG-4)

How to Do It: Lie on your back with your legs straight and crossed at the ankles. Clasp your hands behind your head and execute the Basic Crunch (BLG-1) motion.

Don't Forget: Don't overextend this motion—keep the contraction short and tight.

Alternatives: ILG-3, ILG-5, ILG-6, ILG-7, ILG-8, ILG-9

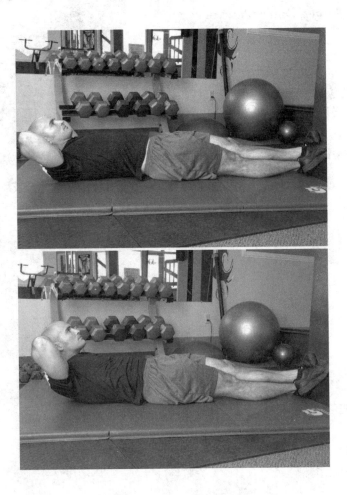

Cross-Body Crunch (ILG-5)

How to Do It: Assume the Basic Crunch (BLG-1) position. Place one hand behind your head and one arm down to your side on the floor. From the side with the hand behind the head, crunch in the direction of your opposite knee, slightly lifting and rolling that side of the head and the shoulders off the floor. Repeat on the other side.

Don't Forget: Don't perform this crunch any differently than the standard motion. Other than having one arm behind your head (instead of two), and slightly crunching across your body instead of directly forward, the rules are the same.

Alternatives: ILG-3, ILG-4, ILG-6, ILG-7, ILG-8, ILG-9

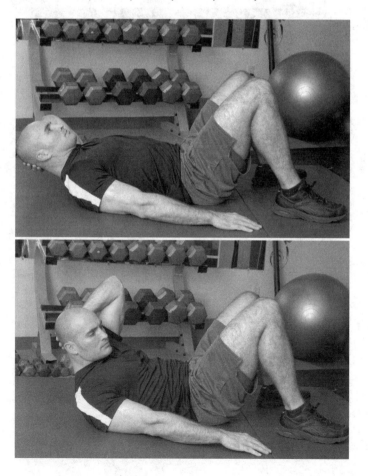

Figure Four Cross-Body Crunch (ILG-6)

How to Do It: This motion is similar to the Cross-Body Crunch (ILG-5). However, instead of having your feet on the floor, you cross one foot over the knee of the opposite leg (figure four position), and lift both feet off the ground. From this position, crunch your head and shoulders, rolling in the direction of your opposite knee. Repeat on the other side.

Don't Forget: Don't allow your legs to drop and then roll up as your execute this motion. Keep your lower body stable, only slightly lifting your hips as you crunch.

Alternatives: ILG-3, ILG-4, ILG-5, ILG-7, ILG-8, ILG-9

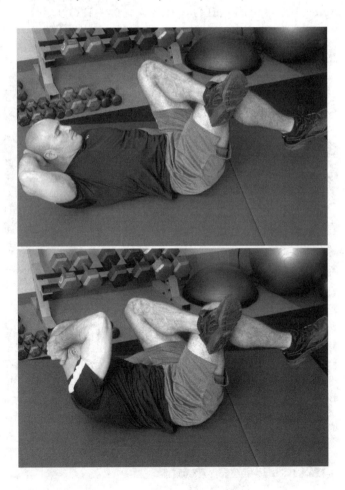

Arms Overhead Crunch (ILG-7)

How to Do It: From the Basic Crunch (BLG-1) position, clasp your hands and extend your arms back and over your head. Holding your arms in that position, roll your head and shoulders off the floor and press your lower back into the floor.

Don't Forget: Don't allow your arms to move forward as your crunch—keep them fixed and stationary in the same plane as your head and neck.

Alternatives: ILG-3, ILG-4, ILG-5, ILG-6, ILG-8, ILG-9

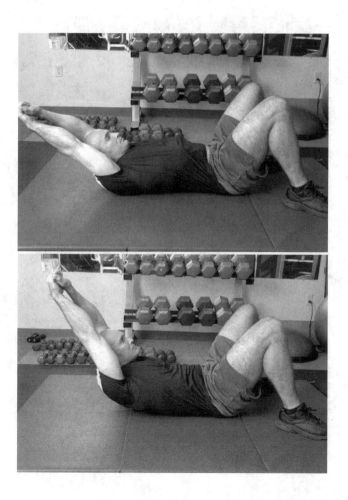

Pulse Crunch (ILG-8)

How to Do It: This crunch starts from the same position as the Basic Crunch (BLG-1). Roll your head and shoulders off the mat to the complete crunch position. Then, limit your return range of motion to approximately half that of a typical crunch, keeping the motion very short and tight.

Don't Forget: Don't execute this motion too quick. Though the exercise is shorter, still maintain control and tempo.

Alternatives: ILG-3, ILG-4, ILG-5, ILG-6, ILG-7, ILG-9

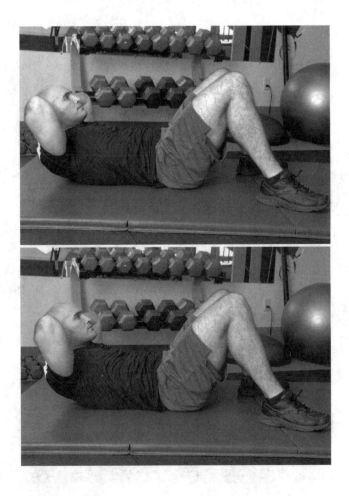

Reach-Through Pulse Crunch (ILG-9)

How to Do It: Place yourself in the Basic Crunch (BLG-1) position. Clasp your hands and extend your arms over your midsection. Crunch to a fully contracted position, then lower yourself approximately half the range of a Basic Crunch. Return and repeat.

Don't Forget: Don't reach through the movement with your shoulders—keep your shoulders and arms locked in position, moving them forward only as far as the crunch range allows.

Alternatives: ILG-3, ILG-4, ILG-5, ILG-6, ILG-7, ILG-8

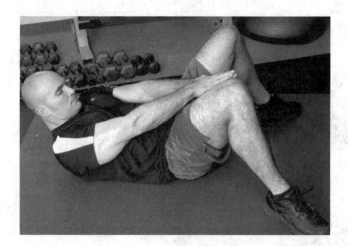

Legs Vertical, Alternate Toe Touch Crunch (ILG-10)

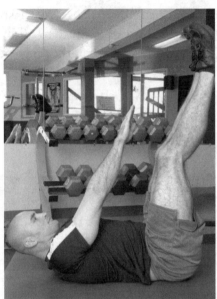

How to Do It: Lie on your back and lift and straighten your legs until they're perpendicular to the floor. Your feet should be positioned slightly narrower than shoulder-width apart. With arms straight and together, crunch up and toward one foot (the motion has a slight twist). Return to the start position and repeat, crunching to the other foot.

Don't Forget: Don't bring your legs toward your hands as you crunch—try to keep them as stationary as possible. Also, don't bend your knees; attempt to keep your legs straight.

Alternatives: ILG-11, ILG-12

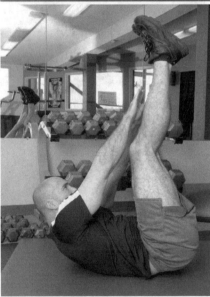

Sumo Stance Alternate Toe Touch (ILG-11)

How to Do It: Lie on your back with your legs straight and raised perpendicular to the floor. From this position, widen your stance, forming a large "V" with your legs. With arms straight and together, crunch up and across your body to one foot, then to the other. Return and repeat.

Don't Forget: Don't simply twist your shoulders. This movement is a variation of a basic crunch—be sure that you're lifting and rolling your head and shoulders up with each repetition.

Alternatives: ILG-10, ILG-12

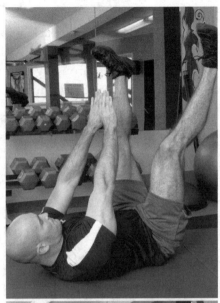

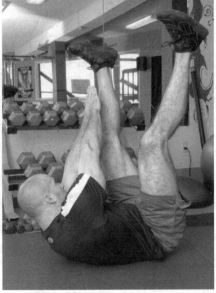

Sumo Stance, Legs Vertical, Reach-Through Crunch (ILG-12)

How to Do It: Lie on your back, with your legs straight, perpendicular to the floor, and forming a large "V." Place your arms together and straight, positioned to reach through your legs. Slowly roll your head and shoulders off the floor, reaching through your legs.

Don't Forget: Don't allow your legs to fall forward toward your head. Keep them stationary and positioned perpendicular to the floor.

Alternatives: ILG-10, ILG-11

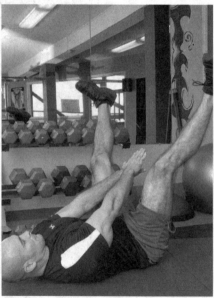 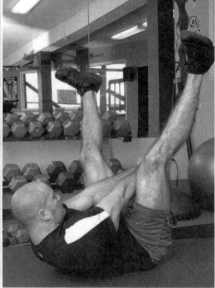

Hip Roll with Lift (ILG-13)

How to Do It: Begin this exercise exactly as the Hip Roll (BLG-13). After rolling the hips, lift and extend your legs upward.

Don't Forget: Don't allow your extended legs to fall back toward your head. Attempt to keep them perpendicular to the floor.

Alternatives: None

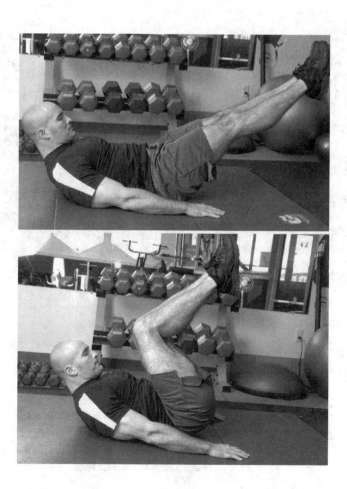

Hip Lift with Twist (ILG-14)

How to Do It: Assume the same position as the Hip Lift (BLG-14). Lift your hips and extend your feet. At the highest point of the motion, rotate and twist your hips, then lower and repeat.

Don't Forget: Don't get sloppy with this exercise. It is a difficult and complex motion that requires concentration and control.

Alternatives: None

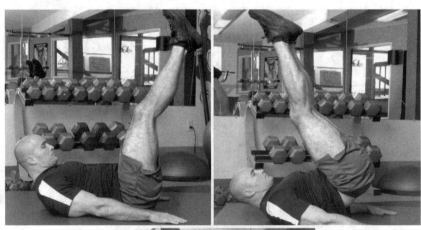

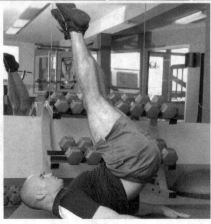

ADVANCED LEVEL GUT (ALG) EXERCISES

These exercises work a large percentage of the muscles that comprise your midsection. These are tough, taxing movements. That's what you want: "simple," "easy," and "sweat-free" don't accurately describe any of these gut exercises. These are movements that make a difference.

Body Plank (ALG-1)

How to Do It: Place yourself on your forearms and toes, with your body suspended and parallel to the floor. Crunch your abdominals by pressing your belly button upwards. Hold this position for a set time period. Rest and repeat.

Don't Forget: Don't allow your lower back to sag toward the floor. Keep your abdominals tight and contracted.

Alternatives: None

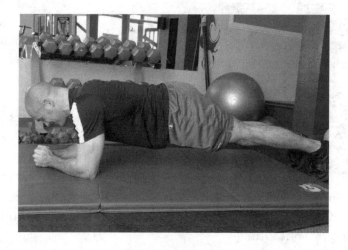

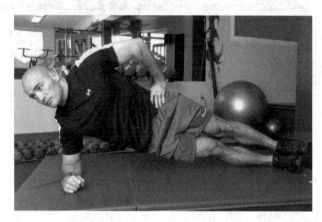

Side Plank (ALG-2)

How to Do It: Resting on your forearm, place your body in a straight line. Your knee, hip, and heels should be in alignment. Hold this position, then rest and repeat. Repeat on the other side.

Don't Forget: Don't allow you hip to sag toward the floor. Work hard to maintain your body in a straight line by keeping all of your gut muscles tight and contracted.

Alternatives: None

Side Plank with Hip Raise (ALG-3)

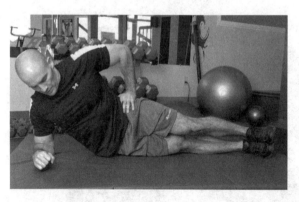

How to Do It: Place yourself in the position of the Side Plank (ALG-2). Lower your hip until it touches the floor, then raise, and repeat. As with the side plank, maintain as straight a line with your body as possible.

Don't Forget: Don't necessarily worry about trying to not touch your free hand to the floor. If necessary, use it to stabilize your position, thus maintaining your form.

Alternatives: ALG-4

Pretzel (ALG-4)

How to Do It: Lie on your side. Bend the bottom leg toward the rear until it is at approximately 90 degrees. The top leg should remain straight and motionless, and both knees should be in alignment with one another. Your free arm should be straight and positioned slightly behind your torso, pointing toward the heel of the bent knee. Slowly crunch your free shoulder and arm toward your heel. Touch your heel with your hand, then lower and repeat. Repeat on the other side.

Don't Forget: Don't become frustrated with the execution of this movement. It initially seems somewhat complex and confusing. However, once mastered, it is an effective side motion.

Alternatives: ALG-3

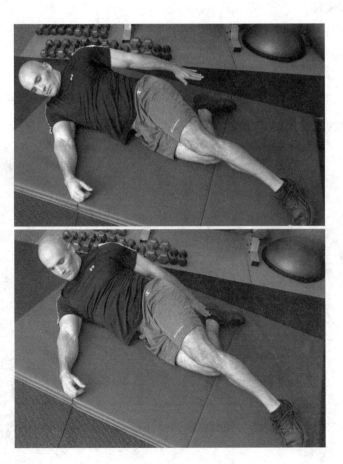

Jack Knife (ALG-5)

How to Do It: Lying on your back, extend your arms straight over your head, approximately twelve inches off the floor. Straighten your legs and hold no less than twelve inches from the floor. Then, slowly bring your arms forward, rolling your head and shoulders off the floor into a crunch position. Simultaneously raise your legs taking care to keep them straight. Touch your hands to your shins or toes, then return and repeat.

Don't Forget: Don't overextend either your arms or your legs to the floor—lowering your legs and arms too close to the floor may make it difficult to keep your lower back from being overarched. Try to maintain contact between your lower back and the floor throughout the motion. Lower your legs and arms only as much as it is still possible to keep your lower back in this position.

Alternatives: ALG-6, ALG-7

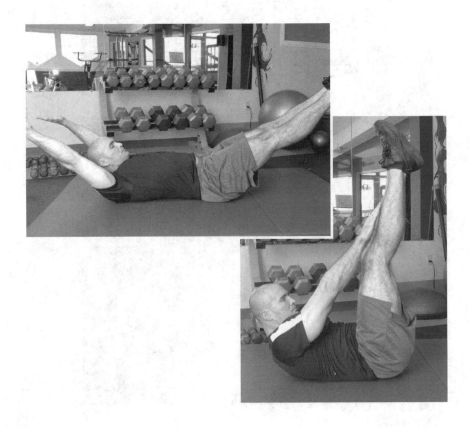

Alternating Jack Knife (ALG-6)

How to Do It: Position yourself exactly as if you're performing the standard Jack Knife (ALG-5). However, instead of lifting both legs simultaneously, alternate your legs, raising each one individually.

Don't Forget: Don't drop your legs—maintain the position of the leg not being lifted at approximately twelve inches off the floor. Keep your lower back pressed into the floor.

Alternatives: ALG-5, ALG-7

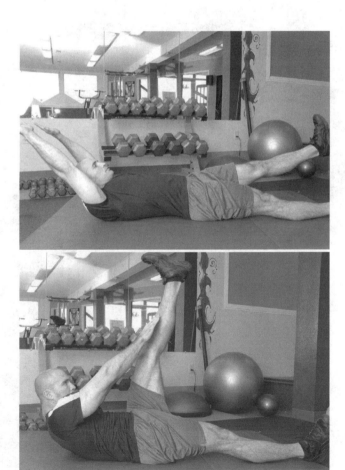

Jack Knife with Legs Crossed and Side Reach (ALG-7)

HOW: Lie on your back with your arms straight and extended over your head. Cross your legs at the ankle, extend, and hold them approximately twelve inches off the floor. With legs crossed at the ankles and arms extended over your head, perform a Jack Knife (ALG-5) motion. However, instead of reaching for your ankles, reach and twist across your body past your shins.

Don't Forget: Don't allow your body to rock excessively side-to-side during the motion. Maintain control.

Alternatives: ALG-5, ALG-6

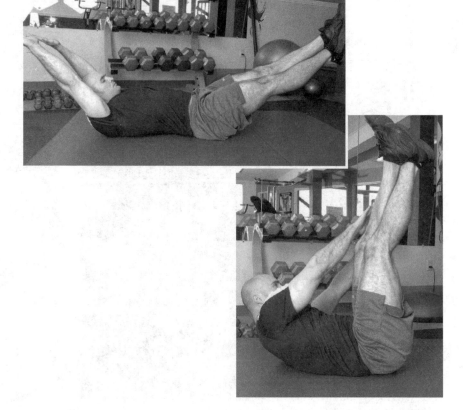

Combination Crunch and Hip Crunch (ALG-8)

How to Do It: Lie on your back with your hands clasped behind your head. Keep your chin up and your elbows pressed back and out. Cross your legs at the ankles, bend your knees, and lift them off the floor. Roll your head and shoulders off the floor and simultaneously lift and roll your hips toward your head.

Don't Forget: Don't over-lift your hips. The lower body motion of this movement should be short and controlled.

Alternatives: ALG-9

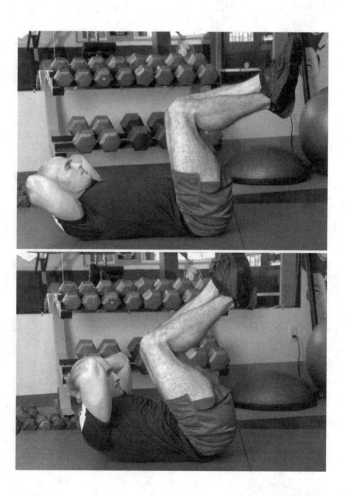

Combination Crunch and Hip Roll (ALG-9)

How to Do It: This motion is almost exactly like the Combination Crunch and Hip Crunch (ALG-8), except instead of keeping your legs raised and crossed, they'll be extended. With legs extended and approximately twelve inches off the floor, slowly pull your knees toward your upper body, rolling your hips off the floor. At the same time, perform a basic crunch motion with your upper body.

Don't Forget: Don't pull your knees to your chest too quickly. Maintain control and don't allow yourself to utilize momentum to complete the exercise.

Alternatives: ALG-8

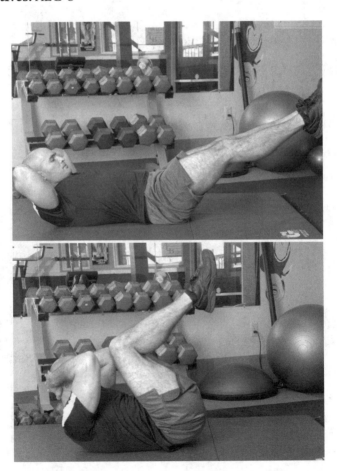

Pilates 100 (ALG-10)

How to Do It: This motion involves holding the abdominals in a contracted position for a predetermined length of time. Lying on your back, roll your head and shoulders off the floor. Place your legs straight and stationary at 12–24 inches off the floor. Holding both your legs and your upper body in place, move your arms up and down slowly while maintaining their position straight and at your side. After pumping your arms 100 times, stop, rest, and repeat.

Don't Forget: Don't allow your upper or lower body to move—keep your entire body absolutely stationary.

Alternatives: None

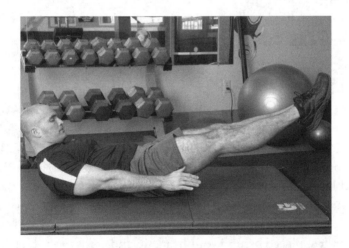

Bicycles (ALG-11)

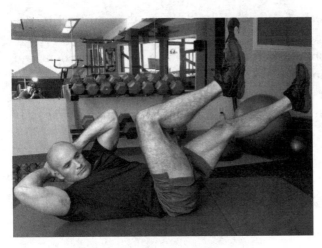

How to Do It: Lie on your back and clasp your hands behind your head. Like the Basic Crunch (BLG-1) and all its variations, keep your elbows out and your chin up. Legs are straight, extended, and off the floor. Alternating sides, roll your head and shoulders off the floor, pulling your opposite knee toward your elbow.

Don't Forget: Don't necessarily touch your elbow to your knee—do so only if your mechanics allow and you are able to maintain proper form.

Alternatives: ALG-12

Single-Side Bicycles (ALG-12)

How to Do It: Position yourself as if performing the Bicycle (ALG-11) exercise. Bend one knee and pull it off the floor as if positioning yourself for the movement. However, the other leg should be either lying flat and straight on the floor or bent with your foot resting on the floor. Place the arm and hand opposite of the elevated leg, behind your head. Keep the elbow out and your chin up. The other arm should be stationary and on the floor beside you. Slowly roll your head and shoulder from the side with your arm placed behind your head, up and across your body toward the elevated knee. As you do this, bring your opposite knee toward your elbow. Return and repeat. Then, repeat on the other side.

Don't Forget: Don't flap your arm—the arm placed behind your head should be stationary throughout the movement.

Alternatives: ALG-11

Supine Sit-Up (ALG-13)

How to Do It: Lie on your back with your legs straight and on the floor. Starting with arms extended over your head, bring your arms forward slowly and with control, rolling your head, shoulders, and entire torso off the floor. Continue rolling forward until you touch your shins.

Don't Forget: Don't raise your hips at any time during the motion—keep your hips and legs securely in place.

Alternatives: ALG-14, ALG-15, ALG-16, ALG-17

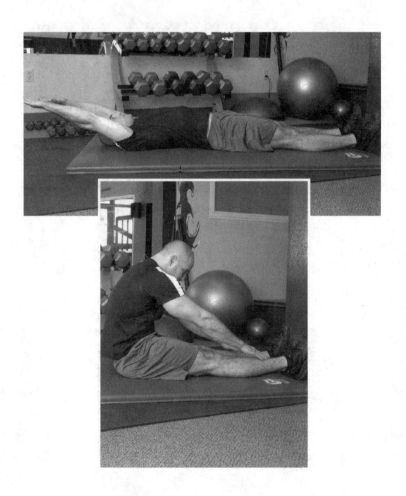

Feet Anchored, Hands Overhead Sit-Up (ALG-14)

How to Do It: Place your feet flat on the ground with knees bent. Extend your arms over your head. Slowly bring your arms forward rolling your head, shoulders, and entire torso off the ground.

Don't Forget: Don't allow your feet to come off the ground. Keep your center of gravity over your hips and maintain your balance.

Alternatives: ALG-13, ALG-15, ALG-16, ALG-17

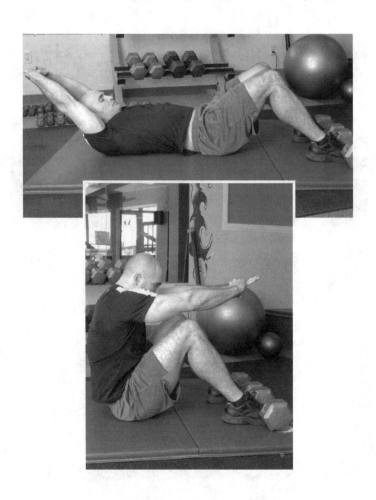

Feet Anchored, Hands on Chest Sit-Up (ALG-15)

How to Do It: Place your feet under an object that can keep your lower body secure and unmoving. Fold your arms and hands over your chest in the "mummy" position. Roll your torso up and off the ground until your chest touches your thighs

Don't Forget: Don't bounce your lower back into the ground in an attempt to begin the exercise by generating momentum. Instead, slowly crunch your head and shoulders up first, followed by lifting your torso to your thighs.

Alternatives: ALG-13, ALG-14, ALG-16, ALG-17

Feet Anchored Sit-Up (ALG-16)

How to Do It: Place your feet under an object that can keep your lower body secure and unmoving. Clasp your hands behind your head. Keeping your chin up and elbows out, roll your torso up and off the ground until your chest touches your thighs.

Don't Forget: Don't pull on your head. Rest your hands behind your head with your chin up. Don't allow your elbows to travel forward while executing the movement.

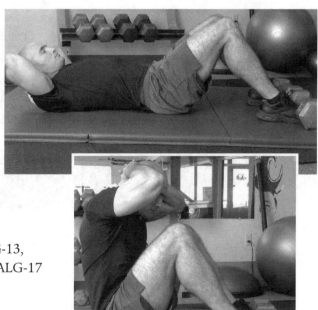

Alternatives: ALG-13, ALG-14, ALG-15, ALG-17

Feet Anchored Sit-Up with Twist (ALG-17)

How to Do It: Perform this motion exactly as if performing the Feet Anchored Sit-Up (ALG-16). However, instead of bringing your upper body straight up, twist your torso and your elbow to the opposite knee. Return and repeat to the other side.

Don't Forget: Don't twist too quickly. The rotation of your torso should coincide with the raising of your torso. Make sure the motion is slow, deliberate, and controlled.

Alternatives: ALG-13, ALG-14, ALG-15, ALG-16

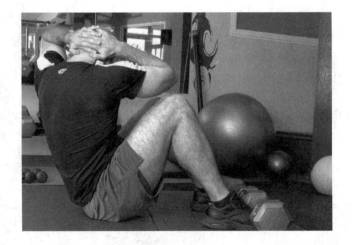

Russian Twist (ALG-18)

How to Do It: Sit on your hips, lean your torso slightly back, and raise your legs off the floor and cross them at the ankles. Your knees should be somewhat bent. Either clasp your hands over your lower chest or hold them 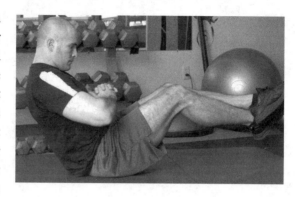 against one another. Keep your elbows up and away from your body. Tighten your abdominals and press your belly button down. From this position, slowly twist at the waist, rotating your upper body. Keep your hips as motionless as possible.

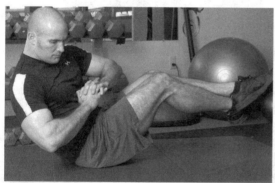

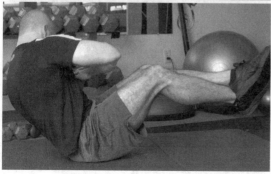

Don't Forget: Don't rotate at the shoulders. Imagine a line emanating from your belly button—be sure the line is moving through the furthest range possible from side to side. This ensures the rotation is occurring at the waist and not further up your torso.

Alternatives: ALG-19, ALG-18A, ALG-18B, ALG-18C

Russian Twist Arms Extended (ALG-19)

How to Do It: Perform this motion exactly as if doing the Russian Twist (ALG-18). However, instead of clasping your hands over your lower chest, your arms should be straight out from your body. The formation of your upper body should resemble the letter "T".

Don't Forget: Don't lose your balance. The arms extended variation of this movement makes maintaining your balance more difficult. Adjust your body position accordingly.

Alternatives: ALG-18

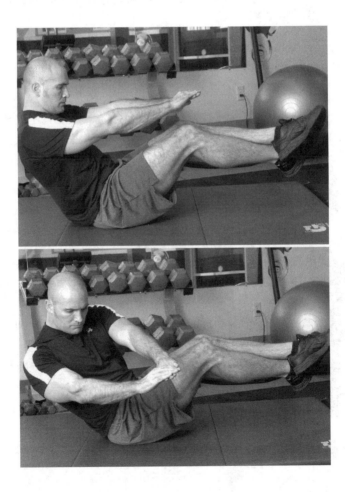

Pike to Plank (ALG-20)

How to Do It: Extend your body in a straight line while face down, supported by your forearms and toes. Slowly raise your hips 3–6 inches upward, crunching your abdominals as your lift. Lower and repeat.

Don't Forget: Don't merely lift your hips. Slowly crunch your abdominals and press your hips upward.

Alternatives: None

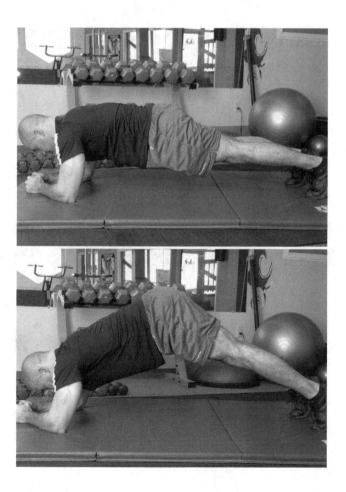

Arms at Side, Legs Bent V-Ups (ALG-21)

How to Do It: Lie on your back with your legs straight and arms at your sides. Simultaneously pull your knees up and raise your torso. Slightly raise your arms for balance and reach toward your legs. When your knees meet your chest, then lower and repeat.

Don't Forget: Don't allow yourself to simply fall to the floor without control—try to lower yourself at the same speed and pace as you raised up.

Alternatives: None

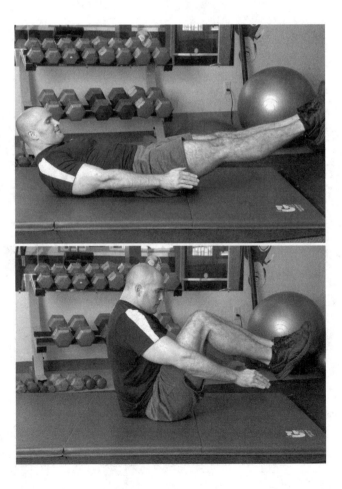

Chapter 6

MAINTAINING YOUR NEW BUTT AND GUT

"How use doth breed a habit in a man!"

—WILLIAM SHAKESPEARE (1564–1616)

IF YOU STARTED THE BUTT & GUT PROGRAM with the idea that it would last 120 days and then end, think again. As I've said, the Butt & Gut Program is your introduction to the lifestyle of health and fitness. It's your "starter kit" to getting off your ass and staying off it. The first 120 days acts merely as your fuse—you're in the race now and it's time to run!

On completing the Butt & Gut Program, take two weeks off. That's right—take two weeks off. I still want you to practice good eating choices, but give your body a much-deserved rest. Rest and recovery time from regular exercise is as much a part of a upholding a successful health and fitness lifestyle as performing the workouts themselves. Taking time off gives your body the rest it needs to continue the physical changes that you're seeking. Don't mistake time off for quitting. It's far from it. Schedule your time away from exercise in the same way that you schedule your time for it. Your time off is an integral part of an exercise program. A good rule of thumb is to take a two-week vacation from exercise for every four months that you exercise.

Second, begin exercising again. Start the Butt & Gut Program over. How? Change the exercises but not the format. Select different movements and, just as before, give yourself optional exercises. Pick one beginning level, one intermediate level, and one advanced level movement for each workout. Perform them in that same sequence: start with the beginning movement and progress to the advanced one. Give yourself as much variety as you'd like with your selections and change the exercises often. Pick three butt exercises and three gut exercises, then use the same set and repetition scheme and progress through the program just as you did the first time.

Third, add different cardiovascular exercises. Learn to incorporate different forms of cardiovascular training, which will keep you mentally fresh and it has the added benefit of making you a more complete athlete. (Yes, athlete.) Incorporate three or more forms of cardiovascular training. Brisk walking and stairs are two that I'd obviously recommend. But going outside isn't always convenient or practical, so having a piece of indoor cardiovascular equipment can be helpful. I am a fan of the elliptical motion machines, and specifically the Precor brand. Precor was the innovator of the idea and have provided the standard by which all others are measured.

Jumping rope is another form of cardiovascular training. It isn't something you see people doing often, but they should—it needs almost no space, no monetary investment, and little training. Jumping rope, however, is tough and after completing twenty minutes, you'll know you've been in a fight. Complete your rope jumping in blocks of time. For instance, start with two minutes, rest and then complete another two minutes. Repeat that sequence until you've reached a total of twenty minutes.

The weather isn't always cooperative, but outside bike riding is also an excellent form of cardiovascular conditioning. Cycling, like stairs, is also easier on your joints than traditional running or jogging. Bike riding is effective, but be sure to ride with purpose and intensity. It's rather easy to take a "Sunday ride" around the neighborhood for twenty minutes, but it's not as effective for improving your conditioning. If you choose cycling, don't be lazy.

Fourth, continue learning about and exploring better nutrition. Variety in your nutrition is as important as variety in your training. Learn to cook with and use different spices. Despite what you may think, deep-fat-fried is not a flavor—it's an unhealthy cooking method, covering the taste of what you're consuming and contributing to your ever-expanding waist line. Grill, season, and marinate—that is, really cook.

Finally, explore other options for your new healthy lifestyle. Take a yoga or Pilates class, hike a mountain, or swim laps at a pool. Get out there and do something. You'll never regret feeling better. Exercise! What are you waiting for?

Continuing the Butt & Gut Program

- Take two weeks off!
- Start the Butt & Gut Program again
- Add more exercises and more variety
- Continue your healthier eating pattern
- Enlarge your "toolbox" of cardiovascular training
- Explore other healthy lifestyle options!

"You gain strength, courage and confidence by every experience in which you really stop to look fear in the face. You are able to say to yourself, 'I have lived through this horror. I can take the next thing that comes along.' You must do the thing you think you cannot do."

—ELEANOR ROOSEVELT (1884–1962)

Butt & Gut Success Stories—
The Cream Rises to the Top

I asked the following warriors to do what they'd never done—change their eating habits and establish better food choices and exercise six days a week. I asked them to do this regardless of rain or shine, schedules, or jobs. I asked them to set their sails and their course for uncharted seas, to take a risk. They learned to trust in themselves and even get a little uncomfortable, because change means getting outside your "little box" and testing some boundaries. These people did just that.

I am proud of the following individuals, because losing weight is hard work. Whether it be five pounds or fifty, the needs are the same—dedication, discipline, and consistency. Old habits die hard and put up one hell of a fight. However, these warriors were up to the challenge, and you are capable of the same thing. Here are their stories.

Deneen

As an overweight, out of shape, stressed-out 38-year-old wife and mother, I knew something in my life had to change. I struggled with finding time to fit more into my already hectic schedule. However, I knew I needed to make some positive health changes in my life if I wanted to be around in the future. I was tired of the excess fat on my body and even more tired of buying larger clothes when I really wanted to purchase smaller ones. When I found out that Marty was looking for people to test his program, I literally begged him to accept me as one of the participants. I just knew I could find twenty minutes in each day for myself, do the workout, and get into shape again.

During the first few weeks, planning the meals proved to be a bit challenging. With the help of a food counting book and several websites that assisted with nutritional data, I gradually eased into the dietary routine. In fact, I made a game of seeing how close I could get to my daily caloric requirements of protein, carbohydrates, and fat. Keeping a daily log of every meal and snack was critical to keeping me on track with the nutritional portion of this program. I carried a little notebook in my purse and kept track of everything that went into my mouth. Every day, I looked up the nutritional breakdown of various foods and recorded them, since I had never counted calories before in my life.

From the beginning, the exercises, coupled with the walking, were precisely the jumpstart I needed to get me off my butt and back in motion. I loved the fact that within twenty minutes I was done with my exercising! The exercises were easy in the beginning of the program and gradually became more challenging, which was perfect for me since I was so out of shape. After the first thirty days, I lost three pounds of fat and almost three inches in my waist and hips. Since I experienced decent results with what I considered to be relatively little effort, I was hooked!

Following Marty's instructions was so easy and yielded such quick results that I could not stop—I was motivated!

Month by month, the exercises and walking/stairs became more challenging, but I never felt discouraged because I knew that I only had to complete a twenty-minute workout each day and *anyone* could do that! I had to work on a mental block where lunges are concerned, though. Lunges are my least favorite exercise, but they do afford some of the best results for shaping your butt and legs. I never came to *love* lunges, but I tolerated them in order to get to the next phase of the program. Initially, I was concerned about walking stairs for twenty minutes; however, the method of gradually working up to twenty minutes of stairs made it a lot easier.

The beauty of this program is that it can be done anywhere, at any time, and by anyone, regardless of fitness level. I performed the exercises in my living room, which was very convenient for me. When I began the walking program, I walked the country roads near my house or in town on my lunch break. My children often walked with me or rode their bicycles to keep me company. This was great because we were spending quality time together and they saw me as a role model for not just "talking the talk" but for actually "walking the walk" of health. As I began to incorporate stairs into my routine, our high school football stadium was the perfect place. I also had access to a "stepmill" at work. The result: I have great calf muscles, my buns are firmer and my legs more toned, and my cardio endurance has increased. I can keep up with the kids now!

Seeing results for the effort I put forth was rewarding and encouraged me to do even better the next month. By the time I got through the program, I had lost 15 pounds of fat, felt great, and looked terrific. I had dropped nearly two pant sizes and received numerous compliments as well as inquiries as to what I had been doing to lose weight. Of course, I shared my "secret" with everyone who would listen. Do I still have room for improvement? You bet I do, but the Butt and Gut Program got me off to a great start. In this fast-paced world in which we live, most people do not take time for themselves. I've only got one life and I have to live it to the fullest, every day.

Emilie

My hips and butt are definitely my problem areas and I'm always looking for something that will "slim" down those areas—usually that means buying the right kind of pants for my shape. I was very excited about Marty's program and liked it even more when I found out it was just a twenty-minute-a-day commitment. I could do twenty minutes a day and I could do this on my own time in my own home with no tapes and no weights.

When I first started the program, it seemed very easy and I wasn't completely convinced that I was really going to see any changes. It didn't seem challenging and I wasn't feeling the results. But I am so glad it started that way—it was a great way to get my body ready to work harder and prepare for the changes that would soon be coming. A couple of weeks of fairly easy workouts and walking got my system ready to accept the stairs work that would soon be coming.

The exercises were simple and once you saw how to do them, you didn't need any further explanation. I could see it once and I was ready to go for that set of exercises. And they can be done anywhere: you can go on vacation and still find the space and the few minutes needed to get this workout done.

My favorite exercises were those that dealt with the abdominal muscles, because those were the ones that I could really see results with. I could feel my stomach becoming tighter and stronger. I could feel my core get stronger and found myself standing up straighter and feeling better about myself. I would always buy shirts that were a little longer to hide my "tummy," but now I tuck in my shirts and wear a belt, not only as an accessory but because I need to!

I spent a week at home with my family and was given many compliments on how great I looked. I had only been working for six weeks and already people could see changes. By that time, I had dropped one pant size and was feeling great. Even on the trip I still had time to do the workouts and I chose to eat well (most of the time). When I came back home, I hadn't regained any weight and that really kept me motivated.

I recently found a pair of jeans packed away in my closet that I had not worn since I was a sophomore in college, roughly four years ago. I

tried them on, fully prepared to not get them past my hips. To my surprise and utter delight, they fit and I didn't have to suck it in at all! I feel
better about myself, stronger and more confident. And it's easy to keep
doing the program. I have found a new and better way to eat and it's not
as difficult as some might think it is. The compliments I get and the way
I look in the mirror are true testaments about how easy it is to lose your
butt and gut if you truly want to. It's not complicated, but it requires dedication. It is not an easy change and not a quick transformation, but the
effects are long lasting and life-changing.

Jillian

I have been obese for about ten years now. I have tried many diets during
that time and have failed to lose weight, mainly because I was looking for
a quick fix. When I didn't see the weight drop off quickly enough, I would
give up. Before I even started a new diet, I knew I would fail. Why?
Because I know that diets don't work in the first place—I needed to
change my whole lifestyle. I've tried to change my activity level a few times
over the years, but unfortunately I gave up when the going got tough. A
major obstacle I had was a negative "inner dialogue," repeatedly telling
myself that I just couldn't do it. I couldn't lose weight, couldn't exercise
regularly, couldn't eat healthy

Marty was the first person who told me straightforwardly with no
fluff that the reason I was fat was because I needed to "get off my ass." He
was right. I lived a sedentary lifestyle: I worked from home and sit in front
of my computer for eight to ten hours a day. When I was done working, I
would sit in front of the television most of the evening. My exercise was
limited to the walk to and from my car and walking around the grocery
store about once a week. When Marty first told me about the Butt & Gut
Program, I knew I had to get involved. I couldn't wait to start! I prepared
myself mentally and emotionally (as much as I could) to let go of what I
call my "crutches"—junk food, watching TV for hours a day, my self-
destructive inner dialogue, all of it.

The first few days went by quickly. I had motivation, self-control, and
a positive attitude—you could say that I was at my emotional and mental

peak. The nutrition part of the program was surprisingly easy for me. My cravings weren't bad at all and the chocolate-lover in me was pacified by the chocolate protein drink I consumed daily. I enjoyed eating healthy and my body loved me for it. I felt alert and had plenty of energy. One of the most important things I learned was that you don't have to starve yourself to lose weight. I eat four to six small meals a day and feel full most of the time. I learned to practice portion control and that you don't have to count calories if you eat the right foods.

The exercises were also relatively easy. Sometimes it was difficult adjusting to a new workout, but I remained steadfast and was feeling awesome! The best part about the exercises is the fact that you only have to work out for twenty minutes a day! Anyone can fit that into his or her schedule. Even when I am away on business, I can do these exercises in my hotel room.

As the fourth week of the program was ending, I started to have some trouble. I was still doing great with the nutrition, but the exercise part of the program was, frankly, kicking my butt! The exercises were getting harder each week and it was tough for me to remain consistent. I skipped a few workouts, always telling myself I had a good reason (which was never reason enough) and the skipped workouts made it harder to get back on track. I was also having trouble with another obstacle for me— not letting myself give up. It used to be so easy for me to just go back to my couch potato life. Marty taught me that I need to expect more of myself than that. My health is one of the most important things in my life and I refused to live my life as a spectator. Marty encouraged me ("consistency, consistency, consistency!" he always says) and soon I was back on course.

Soon, I was beginning to see my body change inside and out—I was losing weight, dropping inches, and had more energy than I have had in years. One night during the second half of the program, my husband asked if I wanted to go for a walk. Normally, I would have come up with some excuse not to go, but on this night I said I'd be glad to join him. He was surprised because I had already done my workout for the day. For me, this night marked a profound change in my life because I realized I was successfully changing my lifestyle. I wasn't just "dieting" or even just following Marty's program—what I realized that night is it's also about making a lifestyle change. To do little things, like putting away the leaf blower and actually raking the leaves myself, or parking the car at the far end of the lot when I go shopping, or walking the tenth of a mile down our easement to get the mail, or walking with my husband, just because.

I have for the most part maintained a healthy, active lifestyle. I am still on the program: I work out twenty minutes a day and eat right. I do slip every now and then, but I have learned that it's okay. I am human and not perfect. Marty taught me that the most important thing is consistency—you have to wake up every morning and make a new decision that you are going to eat right, exercise, and keep your inner dialogue uplifting and positive. Don't beat yourself up or moan and groan while you go through the motions. You need to maintain a healthy, active lifestyle in order to have a longer, happier life! Marty's program will help you achieve these goals.

> *"It's not that some people have willpower and some don't.*
> *It's that some people are ready to change and others are not."*
> —JAMES GORDON, M.D.

Butt & Gut Failures—Dust Off Your Knees!

I started the Butt & Gut Program with twenty-five original participants. The youngest of the group was a woman in her early twenties and the oldest were in their late fifties. The group was comprised of twenty-three women and two men. Participants lived in New York, Oregon, Wisconsin, Kansas, Florida, Missouri, and California. Careers and jobs varied, but this was mainly a "bread-and-butter" middle-class group of baby boomers. A perfect assembly of ready and willing warriors.

It had always been my intent to "spin" any Butt & Gut Program failures into positive contributions to *Busting Your Butt and Gut*. Every weight loss book celebrates successes, but how many openly admonish their failures? None. We can learn a lot from success, but there is also much we can learn from failure.

None of the participants in the Butt & Gut Program could have any good excuses. After all, every thirty days I provided them with a DVD of me performing the exercises exactly as they were supposed to. They were told precisely how many repetitions and how many sets to do. I them how to adapt and adjust and I made myself available by both phone and e-mail. They were told everything they needed to know. How could anyone not succeed? It was my hope that those who didn't complete the program would provide some unique views of their experience and offer explanations for why they were unable to finish, perhaps providing a map showing the potential pitfalls, dead-ends, and obstacles. The Butt & Gut Program failures could offer the means for others to have success, helping them successfully navigate the treacherous seas of establishing the health and fitness lifestyle.

Right out of the gate, I lost about half of those who had committed to the program. Why? I wish I knew: I didn't get one definitive, articulated reason or excuse. Half just simply never even got to the start line and offered no explanation. However, I suspect for many people that superficial commitment is easy. Simply saying "yes" to a program that could potentially change your life involves no investment. Individuals have nothing to lose, that is until the "rubber hits the road." I lost fourteen participants before anyone even broke a sweat.

So, I was left with eleven women and one man. They seemed committed and motivated, but as I suspected, and is usually the case, the group thinned quickly. These individuals were generally middle-aged couch potatoes, with little or no exercise experience, terrible eating habits, and overweight. That's not unusual—that description roughly applies to about 80 percent of the United States population. It is not an understatement to say change for this group will be difficult.

By the end of the first thirty days, the group had dwindled once again, leaving me with seven women and one man, who seemed up for the challenge and ready to press ahead. Though disappointed, I was also again not surprised. Even when we implement what we know are positive changes in our lives, it doesn't necessarily make them any easier to accomplish. Change is hard.

Toward the end of the ninety-day mark of the program, it was obvious to me that I had lost a few more participants: e-mails weren't being returned and communication was sporadic. I knew a few more brave souls were losing yet another battle. With thirty days left and the program's conclusion in sight, only three people remained. Twelve percent of the original group completed the Butt & Gut Program in its entirety. In all honesty, it's about what I expected: my decades of experience in this arena have taught me the difficulties of establishing health and fitness as a lifestyle. I wanted more but I logically knew better.

Change is tough, but the key is to quit looking outside yourself for change, because it isn't there. True change starts from within, and it always does. Quit looking around for all the reasons for your lack of success and start asking yourself why you're making excuses. Most people don't fail to reach their goals—they fail to follow through. Most people simply don't finish because they quit early and a great many hardly get started. I had examples of both with the participants in the original Butt & Gut Program. They justify their choice to stop with excuses, and more often than not their excuses have nothing to do with them, nothing to do with their choices, and nothing to do with decisions they made. Regardless of when it happens however, the result is the same: they quit and thus don't succeed.

> *"To be conscious that you are ignorant*
> *is a great step to knowledge."*
> —BENJAMIN DISRAELI (1804–1881)

Frequently Asked Questions

If I can't exercise first thing in the morning, can I do it in the evening when I get home from work?

Of course. First things first—exercise! Forget about when and where, simply get it done. If your schedule is conducive to working out at 10 P.M., and you'll do it, then exercise at that time. The point is regular, consistent exercise.

I don't have access to enough stairs for the Butt & Gut Program. What could I do as an alternative?

Are you sure? What about where you work—are there stairs in your building? Could you do your stair workout during lunch or a break? What about your parking garage or your apartment complex? If you think about it, there are probably more stairs close to you than you're aware of. However, if there are no stairs to be found, set a treadmill at an 8-degree incline, with a pace of 3.0 to 3.6, and walk.

My knees hurt all the time. How can I do the leg exercises?

Knee pain is a common problem for two reasons: the muscles that surround your knees are weak and you're probably overweight. Your knees are carrying the load of your excesses and lack of exercise. The simple fix is to initially limit the range of motion with the exercises that cause the most discomfort. As you get stronger, then increase the range of motion. With time and effort, your range of motion will improve and your pain will decrease as your muscles become stronger.

I want to eat better, but the taste of low-fat and grilled foods seems so bland to me. What can I do to add flavor?

Chances are that you've eaten high-sugar and high-fat foods for most of your life. You have conditioned your taste buds, and after years of consuming the same foods you become physically and psychologically comfortable with certain tastes and flavors. To some degree, you're an addict. But you can change your eating habits and learn to enjoy new, healthier tastes and flavors. It is not easy, however, and it will take effort and time. Start by experimenting with spices and non-fat flavorings. Challenge yourself to make foods that you'll enjoy.

My husband thinks I look fine the way I am and says that I don't need to lose any weight. He wants the same foods for dinner we've always had.

Of course, he does—your husband is not ready to change. He thinks you look fine the way you are because he wants to keep eating the same "crap" every night. He's not being kind, he's being selfish. You can't force him to begin making the changes that you are—we each have to find our own path. But that doesn't mean you have to cook hamburgers and french fries for him. Tell him he's more than welcome to have whatever he wants—just show him to the kitchen and tell him to have at it.

Being around my co-workers makes changing my lifestyle difficult. Everyone I work with is overweight and out of shape. It's hard to eat a chicken breast and salads while they are eating super burritos.

Yes, it is. It's easy to just fall in rank-and-file with everyone else. Like lambs to the slaughterhouse, most of us just follow along. But where's the value in that? Is this a group you want to copy? Do you want to be fat and out of shape? Aren't you tired of shopping for the latest in "double-wide" fashions? Wouldn't you like to ride a bike with your child without any thought about how far or how difficult the ride might be? Of course, you would. Take pride in being an individual not a follower, and break rank!

I lack the motivation—I can't make myself exercise. What do I do?

This is why I preach establishing habit. Measurable, physical goals alone won't get it done and don't provide the motivation that all the so-called experts say it will. Don't worry about or keep searching for the ever-elusive "motivation." *Just do it!* Get up, get going, and get it done. Quit whining, complaining, and waiting. Do you brush your teeth every morning because you and your dentist set "goals"? No, you brush your teeth so you *don't* have to visit your dentist. Twenty minutes of exercise a day is the best health insurance you'll ever have.

I want to do more cardiovascular training. Can I do stairs every day with my other workouts?

No, this is what's known as the "too much, too soon" trap. Good intentions, sure, but misguided. Don't fill your plate too full because it sets you up for failure. You'll eventually become overwhelmed and overtrained. Remember the tortoise and the hare.

Why can't I just start with the lowest calorie plan that you've suggested?

Because you'll fail: you'll never be able to keep to that drastic of a lifestyle change. Don't even try. Baby steps, my friend, baby steps.

Why aren't there any arm or shoulder exercises in the Butt & Gut Program? The back of my arms are one of my main "problem" areas.

The muscles that comprise the shoulders and arms are relatively small muscles. Spending a great deal of time and effort on small muscles with isolation exercises is one of the biggest mistakes of most exercisers. The Butt & Gut Program focuses on movements that incorporate multiple muscles with compound applications, which means a lot of muscles are worked with one motion. More muscles moving means more calories burned.

Will I have to exercise for the rest of my life?

Yes. Here's a tissue—have a nice cry. Now, pull up your big girl or boy panties, and start busting your butt and gut!

CONCLUSION

*"Twenty years from now, you will be more disappointed
by the things you didn't do than by the ones you did.
So throw off the bowlines. Sail away from the safe harbor.
Catch the trade winds in your sails.
Explore. Dream. Discover."*

—UNKNOWN

SEDENTARY LIFESTYLES ARE HERE to stay—that's a fact. Short of a cataclysmic world disaster, most of us are not going to be foraging for food anytime soon or chasing down dinner with spears and clubs. Desk jobs are here and they're not going anywhere. Do you think that people 100 years ago were any different from you? You think that, if given the choice, our great grandparents wouldn't have rather tapped their fingers on a computer keyboard than plowed the prairie sod? They weren't better than you; they just had fewer choices. We don't plow sod because we don't have to. However, though physical labor is no longer a mainstay of daily existence for most of us, it also isn't an excuse for our current overweight condition.

We have choices. For most of us, a cushy desk chair and trips to the break room comprise most of our day. We drive a car or ride mass transit to work, sit almost all day, then return home and sit all evening in front of the "boob tube" (ever wonder why that label stuck?). Our lives are easy, simple, and pleasant. But our pleasant choices have come with a price and it's a stiff one—your health.

Okay, we're fat, our lifestyles are sedentary, and we eat too much of the wrong stuff. That's the problem. Forget about your chromium levels, your cortisol levels, your thyroid imbalances, your lack of testosterone, your mom's genetics, the bacteria in your colon, and on and on. Forget about all that nonsense. Ninety-nine percent of you suffer from eating too much "crap" and from too much sitting on your ass! It is simple, tough to hear, *and* true.

Here's the good news: you can change today. You can start right now—it's never too late, but it's also never too early. What are you waiting for? What in your life won't be improved by your feeling better? Get out of the passenger seat, grab the wheel, and hit the gas! Start busting your butt and gut!

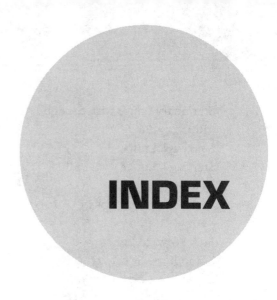

INDEX

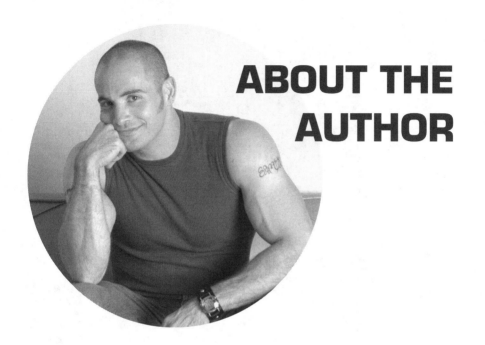

ABOUT THE AUTHOR

Marty Tuley is an author, personal trainer, competitive natural body-builder, and power lifter. He owned and operated a commercial health club for more than ten years. Whether he's training a professional athlete, a homemaker, or a nine-to-fiver, he touts the same exercise message: *It's not about the magic pill or the routine. It's all about dedication, consistency, and plain ole HARD work. Get used to it!*

Marty lives in Lawrence, Kansas, with his wife, Lovena, where they own and operate an exclusive, one-on-one personal-training studio. When they're not at the studio, they're busy spending time with their adopted dogs, Neesha, Blitz, and Bud.

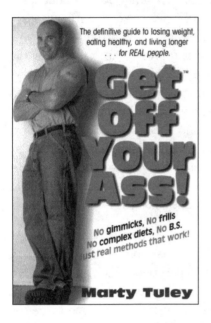

In the first lap, Education, Tuley, with brutal honesty, explores the reasons why the "growing epidemic of obesity" in America has become a cliché. He takes on the fitness industry of which he is a part, breaking down in simple fashion why gyms fail, why most diets are bunk, and why the so-called experts are just plain wrong. Next, he introduces his unorthodox four-month exercise program, which focuses on realistic goals and progress for the exercise novice. The final lap, Nutrition, is chock full of sound, simple advice for eating well. It focuses on teaching the reader a new way of eating and living, not on providing complex, short-term diet solutions or endless lists of "good" and "bad" foods. Tuley even encourages readers to literally smash and batter their scales, a notion that undoubtedly would bring smiles to all those dieters who have spent many frustrating years trying to count calories.

All the while, Tuley candidly challenges readers in a no-nonsense, in-your-face style that forces them to rethink the way they're living. Readers can't help but feel as if they have their own personal coach pushing them every step of the way, doling out praise when they've stayed disciplined and barking in their ear when they've strayed from that road to better health.